HEALTH AND HEALING
IN YOGA

HEALTH AND HEALING
IN YOGA

SELECTIONS FROM
THE WRITINGS AND TALKS OF
THE MOTHER

SRI AUROBINDO ASHRAM
PONDICHERRY

First edition 1979
Eighth impression 2003

Price Rs. 65.00
ISBN 81-7058-023-4

tment,

Lotus Press
PO Box 325
Twin Lakes, WI 53181 USA
www.lotuspress.com
lotuspress@lotuspress.com

y

Publisher's Note

The extracts for this book have been selected from the writings and talks of the Mother. Most of the chapters begin with a series of short written statements arranged under the first title. The titles which follow are generally longer passages taken from talks; a few are from essays and messages. The talks were given in French, the written material either in French or in English.

A sketch of the Mother's life, a glossary of Sanskrit and philosophical terms, and a list of references to the text have been provided at the end of the book.

Courage! Hearken to the lesson that the rising sun brings to the earth with its first rays each morning. It is a lesson of hope, a message of solace.

You who weep, who suffer and tremble, who dare not expect an end to your ills, an issue to your pangs, behold: there is no night without dawn and the day is about to break when darkness is thickest; there is no mist that the sun does not dispel, no cloud that it does not gild, no tear that it will not dry one day, no storm that is not followed by its shining triumphant bow; there is no snow that it does not melt, nor winter that it does not change into radiant spring. . . .

If ordeal or fault has cast you down, if you have sunk into the nether depths of suffering, do not grieve — for there indeed the divine love and the supreme blessing can reach you! Because you have passed through the crucible of purifying sorrows, the glorious ascents are yours.

—The Mother

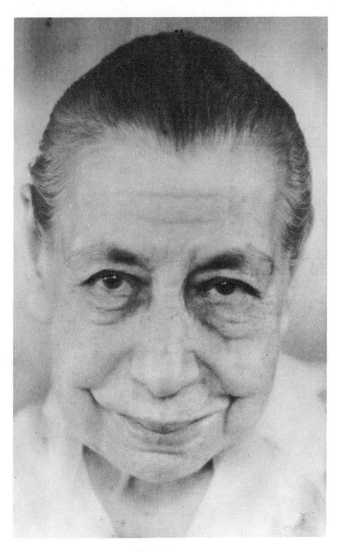

THE MOTHER

CONTENTS

PART IV

THE CYCLE OF LIFE

PART I

CAUSES OF ILLNESS

I

DISEQUILIBRIUM OF THE BEING

Illness: A Disharmony of the Inner Being

Sri Aurobindo says,
   "Disease is needlessly prolonged and ends in death oftener
than is inevitable, because the mind of the patient supports
and dwells upon the disease of the body",
   and I add,
   "An illness of the body is always the outer expression and
translation of a disorder, a disharmony in the inner being;
unless this inner disorder is healed, the outer cure cannot be
total and permanent."

*

Look for the inner causes of disharmony much more than the
outer ones. It is the inside which governs the outside.

*

You ask me whether your illness comes from yoga. By no
means — far from damaging health, yoga helps to build up one
that is robust and unfailing.

Illness: A Break of Equilibrium

I told you the other day that I would speak to you of illness;[1]
I thought of it today and have made notes.... For you may tell

   [1] "Next time we shall speak of health and illness and I shall con-
found all those who are attached by iron chains to their illness and

me there are microbes, and that there are people who have no thought of illness and catch it all the same; but thinking is not the only factor, not by any means. Still, I shall try to explain to you now the notes I have made. (*Mother looks at a paper.*)

I have told you first of all that all illness without any exception — without exception — is the expression of a break in equilibrium. But there are many kinds of breaks in equilibrium.... First, I am speaking only of the body, I am not speaking of the nervous illnesses of the vital or of mental illnesses. We shall see that later on. We are speaking only of this poor little body. And I say that all illnesses, all, whatever they may be (I would add even accidents) come from a break in equilibrium. That is, if all your organs, all the members and parts of your body are in harmony with one another, you are in perfect health. But if there is the slightest imbalance anywhere, immediately you get either just a little ill or quite ill, even very badly ill, or else an accident occurs. That always happens whenever there is an inner imbalance.

But then, to the equilibrium of the body, you must add the equilibrium of the vital and the mind. For you to be able to do all kinds of things with immunity, without any accident happening to you, you must have a triple equilibrium — mental, vital, physical — and not only in each of the parts, but also in the three parts in their mutual relations.... If you have done a little mathematics, you should have been taught how many combinations that makes and what a difficult thing it means! There lies the key to the problem. For the combinations are innumerable, and consequently the causes of illness too are innumerable, the causes of accidents also are innumerable. Still, we are going to try to classify them so that we may understand.

who do not want to let it go! I shall give them scissors to cut their chains."

First of all, from the point of view of the body — just the body — there are two kinds of disequilibrium: functional and organic. I do not know if you are aware of the difference between the two; but you have organs and then you have all the parts of your body: nerves, muscles, bones and all the rest. Now, if an organ by itself is in disequilibrium, it is an organic disequilibrium, and you are told: that organ is ill or perhaps it is badly formed or it is not normal or an accident has occurred to it. But it is the organ that is ill. But the organ may be in a very good condition, all your organs may be in a very good condition, but there is still an illness as they do not function properly: there is a lack of balance in the functioning. You may have a very good stomach, but suddenly something happens to it and it does not function properly; or the body may also be excellent, but something happens to it and it does not work properly any more. Then you have an illness due to functional imbalance not organic imbalance.

Generally, illnesses due to functional imbalance are cured much more quickly and easily than the others. The others become a little more serious. Sometimes they become very grave. So there are already two domains to see and know, but if you have a little knowledge of your body and the habit of observing its working, you can know what kind of imbalance yours is.

Most often when you are young and leading a normal life, the imbalance is purely functional. There are only a few poor people who for one reason or other have had an accident or imbalance before their birth, these carry with them something that is much more difficult to cure (not that it is incurable; in theory, there is nothing incurable), but it becomes more difficult.

Good. Now what are the causes of this imbalance, whatever it may be? As I told you just now, the causes are innumerable;

because, first of all, there are all the inner causes, that is, those personal to you, and then all the external causes, those that come to you from outside. That makes two major categories.

The internal causes:

We said: you have a brain, lungs, a heart, a stomach, a liver, etc. If each one does its duty and works normally and if all move together in harmony at a given moment and in the right way (note that it would be very complicated if you were obliged to think of all that, and I am afraid things would not go right all the time! Fortunately, it does not need our conscious thinking), admitting however they are in good harmony with one another, good friends, in perfect agreement, and each one fulfilling its task, its movement at the right time, in tune with the rest, neither too soon nor too late, neither too fast nor too slow, indeed, every one going all right, then you are marvellously well! Suppose now that one of them, for some reason or other, happens to be in a bad mood: it does not work with the necessary energy, at the required moment it goes awhile on strike. Do not believe that it alone will fall ill: the whole system will go wrong and you will feel altogether unwell. And if, unfortunately, there is a vital imbalance, that is, a disappointment or too violent an emotion or too strong a passion or something else upsetting your vital, that comes in addition. And if furthermore your thoughts roam about and you begin to have dark ideas and formulate frightful things and make catastrophic formations, then after that you are sure to fall ill altogether.... You see the complication, don't you, just a tiny thing can go the wrong way and thus through an inner contagion can lead to something very serious. So what is important is to control things immediately. One must be conscious, conscious of the working of one's organs, aware of the one that does not behave very well, telling it immediately what is to be done to set itself right. What is needed (I shall explain it to you later on) is to give them a lesson as one does to little children. When they begin indulging in unhealthy fancies (indeed it is then the occasion to say it) you must tell them: no, it is not like that the work is to be done, it is the other way! Suppose for example, your heart begins to throb madly; then you must make it calm, you tell it that this is not the way to act, and at the same time (solely to help it) you take in long very regular rhythmic breaths, that is, the lung becomes the mentor of the heart and teaches it how to work properly. And so on. I could give you countless examples.

Good. We say then that there is an imbalance between the different parts of the being, disharmony in their working. That is what I have just told you. And then there are internal conflicts. These are quarrels. There are internal quarrels among the different parts of yourself. Supposing there is an organ (it happens very often) that needs rest and there is another that wants action, and both at the same time. How are you going to manage it? They begin to quarrel. If you do what one wants, the other protests! And so you have to find a middle term to put them in harmony. And then, at times, if you add to the physical the vital and mental (I do not speak of the speculative mind or the independent vital, I am speaking of the mental and vital parts of the *body*, because there is a physical vital and a physical mind; there is a physical mind and this physical mind is the worst of all, it is that which goes on all the time and you have the utmost difficulty in stopping it: it goes on and on and on); well, if there is a dispute between them, between the mind, the vital and the physical, you have a battlefield, and this battlefield can become the cause of all possible illnesses. They fight violently. One wants something, the other does not, they quarrel and you are in a kind of internal whirlwind. That can give you fever — you do get it usually — or else you are seized by an inner shivering and you have no longer any control. For the most important of all causes for bodily illness is that the body begins to get restless; it trembles and the trembling increases more and more, more and more and you feel that you will never be able to re-establish the balance, it eludes you. Then in that case you must know what the dispute is about, the reason of the dispute and find out how to reconcile the people within you.

All these are functional imbalances.

There are other kinds of imbalance and they are more or less a part of what you were saying just now. There is an aspiration within you (I am now speaking of people who do yoga or at any rate know what the spiritual life is and try to walk on the path), within you there is a part of the being — either mental or vital or sometimes even physical — that has understood well, has much aspiration, its special aptitudes, that receives the forces well and is making good progress. And then there are others that cannot, others still that don't want to (that of course is very bad), but there are yet others that want to very much but cannot, do not have the capacity, are not ready. So there is something that rises upward and something that does not move. That causes a terrible imbalance. And usually this translates itself into some illness or other, for you are in such a state of inner tension between something that cannot or something that clings, that does not want to move and something else that wants to: that produces a frightful unease and the result usually is an illness.

Now there is the opposite, almost the opposite, that is, the whole being goes ahead, progresses, advances in an increasing equilibrium and achieves remarkable progress; you have the feeling you are in a wonderfully favourable state, everything is going on well, you are sure; and you see yourself already gloriously well on the way.... Crack! an illness. Then you say: "How is it? I was in such a good condition and now I have fallen ill! It is not fair." But this happens because you are not completely conscious. There was a small part in the being that did not want to move. Usually it is something in the vital; sometimes it is a tiny mental formation that does not agree to follow; sometimes it is simply something in the body which is quite inert or has not the slightest intention of moving, that wants things to remain always as they are. It pulls backward, separates itself wilfully, and naturally, even if it is quite small, it brings about such an imbalance in the being that you fall ill. And then you say to yourself: "It is truly a pity, I was going on so well, it is not fair! Truly God is not kind!... When I was making so much progress, He ought to have prevented me from becoming ill!"... It is like that.

Now, there is still another thing. You do the yoga according to your capacity. You have been told: "Open yourself, you will receive the Force." You have been told: "Have faith, be of goodwill and you will be protected." And indeed you are bathed in the Consciousness, bathed in the Force, bathed in the Protection and to the extent you have faith and open yourself, you receive all that, and it helps you in keeping fit and in rejecting the little inner distrubances and re-establishing order when these come, in protecting yourself against small attacks or accidents which might have happened. But if somewhere in your being — either in your body or even in your vital or mind, either in several parts or even in a single one — there is an incapacity to receive the descending Force, this acts like a grain of sand in a machine. You know, a fine machine working quite well with everything going all right, and you put into it just a little sand (nothing much, only a grain of sand), suddenly everything is damaged and the machine stops. Well, just a little lack of receptivity somewhere, something that is unable to receive the Force, that is completely shut up (when one looks at it, it becomes as it were a little dark spot somewhere, a tiny thing hard as a stone: the Force cannot enter into it, it refuses to receive it — either it cannot or it will not) and immediately that produces a great imbalance; and this thing that was moving upward, that was blooming so wonderfully, finds itself sick, and sometimes just when you were in the normal equilibrium; you were in good health, everything was going on well, you had nothing to complain about. One day when you grasped a new idea, received a new impulse, when you had a great aspiration and received a great force and had a marvellous experience, a beautiful experience opening to you inner doors, giving you a knowledge you did not have before; then you were sure that everything was going to be all right.... The next day, you are taken ill. So you say: "Still that? It is impossible! That should not happen." But it was quite simply what I have just said: a grain of sand. There was something that could not receive; immediately it brings about a disequilibrium. Even though very small it is enough, and you fall ill.

You see there are reasons! — many reasons, numberless reasons. For all these things combine in an extraordinarily complex way, and in order to know, in order to be able to cure an illness, one must find out its cause, not its microbe. For it happens that (excuse me, I hope there are no doctors here!), it happens that when microbes are there, they find out magnificent remedies to kill the microbes, but these remedies cure some and make others much more ill! Nobody knows why.... Perhaps I know why. Because the illness had another cause than the purely physical one; there was another; the first was only an outer expression of a different disorder; and unless you touched that, discovered that disorder, never would you be able to prevent the illness from coming. And to discover the disorder, you must have an extensive occult knowledge and also a deep knowledge of all the inner workings of each one.

Thus we have seen in brief, very rapidly all the internal causes. Now there are external causes that come and bring complications.

If you were in a perfectly harmonious environment where everything was full of a total and perfect goodwill, then evidently you could lay the blame only on yourself. But the difficulties that are within are also without. You can, to a certain extent, establish an inner equilibrium, but you live in surroundings full of imbalance. Unless you shut yourself up in an ivory tower (which is not only difficult but not always recommendable), you are obliged to receive what comes from outside. You give and you receive; you breathe in and absorb. So there is a mixture and that is why one can say that all is contagious, for you live in a state of ceaseless vibrations. You give out your vibrations and receive also the vibrations of others, and these vibrations are of a very complex kind. There are still (we shall say for simplifying the language) mental vibrations, vital vibrations, physical vibrations and many others. You give, you receive; you give, you receive. It is a perpetual play. Even granting that there is no bad will, there is necessarily contagion. And as I was saying just now, all is contagious, everything. You are looking at the effect of an accident: you absorb a certain vibration. And if you are over-sensitive and over and above that you have fear or disgust (which is the same thing, disgust is only a moral expression of a physical fear), the accident can be translated physically in your body. Naturally you will be told that it is persons in a state of nervous imbalance who have such reactions. It is not quite that. They are persons with an ultra-suprasensitive vital, that is all. And it is not always a proof of inferiority, on the contrary! For as you progress spiritually, a certain hypersensitiveness of nerves occurs and if your self-control does not increase along with your sensibility, all kinds of untoward things may happen to you.

But that is not the only thing.

Unhappily there is much bad will in the world; and among the different kinds of bad will there is the small type that comes from ignorance and stupidity, there is the big type that comes from wickedness and there is the formidable one that is the result of anti-divine forces. So, all that is in the atmosphere (I am not telling you this to frighten you, for it is well understood that one should fear nothing — but it is there all the same) and these things attack you, sometimes intentionally, sometimes unintentionally. Unintentionally, through other people: others are attacked, they don't know, they pass it on without even being aware of it. They are the first victims. They pass the illness to others. But there are wilful attacks. We were speaking the other day of mental formations and of wicked people who make mental formations to harm you, make them wilfully to do harm. And then there are others who go still a step further.

There is a misguided, perverted occultism which is called black magic, it is a thing one must never touch. But unfortunately, there are people who touch it through pure wickedness. You must not believe it is an illusion, a superstition: it is real. There are people who know how to do magic and do it, and with their magic they obtain altogether detestable results.... It is understood of course that when you have no fear and remain under protection, you are sheltered. But there is a "when", there is a condition, and then if the condition is not always fulfilled, very unpleasant things may happen. So long as you are in a state full of strength, full of purity — that is, in a state of invincibility, if anybody does anything against you, that falls back upon him automatically, as when you throw a tennis-ball against the wall, it comes back to you; the thing comes back to them exactly in the same way, sometimes with a greater force, and they are punished by the very thing through which they sinned. But naturally it all depends on the person against whom the magic is done, on his inner force and purity.... These things I have known, many cases like this. And in such cases, in order to resist, one must be, as I said, a warrior in the vital, that is, a spiritual fighter in the vital. All who do yoga sincerely must become that, and when they do become that, they are altogether sheltered. But one of the conditions for becoming it is never to have bad will or a bad thought towards others. For if you have a bad feeling or bad will or a bad thought, you come down to their level and when you are on the same level with them, well, you may receive blows from them.

Now, without going to that extreme, there are in the physical atmosphere, the earth-atmosphere, numerous small entities which you do not see, for your sight is too limited, but which move about in your atmosphere. Some of them are quite nice, others very wicked. Generally these little entities are produced by the disintegration of vital beings — they pullulate — and these form quite an unpleasant mass. There are some which do very fine things. I believe I narrated to you the story of the little beings who tugged at my sari to tell me that the milk was about to boil and that I had to go and see that it did not boil over. But all of them are not so good. Some of them like to play ugly little tricks, wicked little pranks. And so most often it is they who are behind an accident. They like little accidents, they like the whole whirl of forces that gather round an accident: a mass of people, you know, it is very amusing! And then that gives them their food, because, in reality, they feed upon human vitality thrown out of the body by emotions and excitements. So they say: just a small accident, it is quite nice, many accidents!...

And then if there is a group of such small entities, they may clash with one another, because among themselves they do not have a very peaceful life: clashing with one another, fighting, destroying, demolishing each other. And that is the origin of microbes. They are forces of disintegration. But they continue to be alive even in their divided forms and this is the origin of germs and microbes. Therefore most microbes have behind them a bad will and that is what makes them so dangerous. And unless one knows the quality and kind of bad will and is capable of acting upon it, there is a ninety-nine per cent chance of not finding the true and total remedy. The microbe is a very material expression of something living in a subtle physical world and that is why these very microbes ... that are always around you, within you, for years together do not make you ill and then suddenly they make you fall ill.

There is another reason. The origin of the microbes and their support lie in a disharmony, in the being's receptivity to the adverse force. I will tell you a story. I do not know whether I have already told it to you, but I am going to tell you now for it will give you an illustration.

I was in Japan. It was at the beginning of January 1919. Anyway, it was the time when a terrible flu raged there in the whole of Japan, which killed hundreds of thousands of people. It was one of those epidemics the like of which is rarely seen. In Tokyo, every day there were hundreds and hundreds of new cases. The disease appeared to take this turn: it lasted three days and on the third day the patient died. And people died in such large numbers that they could not even be cremated, you understand, it was impossible, there were too many of them. Or otherwise, if one did not die on the third day, at the end of seven days one was altogether cured; a little exhausted but all the same completely cured. There was a panic in the town, for epidemics are very rare in Japan. They are a very clean people, very careful and with a fine morale. Illnesses are very rare. But still this came, it came as a catastrophe. There was a terrible fear. For example, people were seen walking about in the streets with a mask on the nose, a mask to purify the air they were breathing, so that it might not be full of the microbes of the illness. It was a common fear.... Now, it so happened I was living with someone who never ceased troubling me: "But what is this disease? What is there behind this disease?" What I was doing, you know, was simply to cover myself with my force, my protection so as not to catch it and I did not think of it any more and continued doing my work. Nothing happened and I was not thinking of it. But constantly I heard: "What is this? Oh, I would like to know what is there behind this illness. But could you not tell me what this illness is, why it is there?..." etc. One day I was called to the other end of the town by a young woman whom I knew and who wished to introduce me to some friends and show me certain things: I do not remember now what exactly was the matter, but anyway I had to cross the whole town in a tram-car. And I was in the tram and seeing these people with masks on their noses, and then there was in the atmosphere this constant fear, and so there came a suggestion to me; I began to ask myself: "Truly, what is this illness? What is there behind this illness? What are the forces that are in this illness?..." I came to the house, I passed an hour there and I returned. And I returned with a terrible fever. I had caught it. It came to you thus, without preparation, instantaneously. Illnesses, generally illnesses from germs and microbes take a few days in the system: they come, there is a little battle inside; you win or you lose, if you lose you catch the illness, it is not complicated. But there, you just receive a letter,

open the envelope, hop! puff! The next minute you have
the fever. Well, that evening I had a terrible fever. The
doctor was called (it was not I who called him), the doctor
was called and he told me: "I must absolutely give you this
medicine." It was one of the best medicines for the fever,
he had just a little (all their stocks were exhausted, everyone
was taking it); he said: "I have still a few packets, I shall
give you some" — "I beg of you, do not give it to me, I won't
take it." He was quite disgusted: "It was no use my coming
here." So I said: "Perhaps it was no use!" And I remained
in my bed, with my fever, a violent fever. All the while I
was asking myself: "What is this illness? Why is it there?
What is there behind it?..." At the end of the second day,
as I was lying all alone, I saw clearly a being, with a part of
the head cut off, in a military uniform (or the remains of a
military uniform) approaching me and suddenly flinging himself upon my chest, with that half a head to suck my force.
I took a good look, then realised that I was about to die. He
was drawing all my life out (for I must tell you that people
were dying of pneumonia in three days). I was completely
nailed to the bed, without movement, in a deep trance. I
could no longer stir and he was pulling. I thought: now it
is the end. Then I called on my occult power, I gave a
big fight and I succeeded in turning him back so that he could
not stay there any longer. And I woke up.

But I had seen. And I had learnt, I had understood that
the illness originated from beings who had been thrown out
of their bodies. I had seen this during the First Great War,
towards its end, when people used to live in trenches and
were killed by bombardment. They were in perfect health,
altogether healthy and in a second they were thrown out of
their bodies, not conscious that they were dead. They did
not know they hadn't a body any more and they tried to find

in others the life they could not find in themselves. That is, they were turned into so many countless vampires. And they vampirised upon men. And then over and above that, there was a decomposition of the vital forces of people who fell ill and died. One lived in a kind of sticky and thick cloud made up of all that. And so those who took in this cloud fell ill and usually got cured, but those who were attacked by a being of that kind invariably died, they could not resist. I know how much knowledge and force were necessary for me to resist. It was irresistible. That is, if they were attacked by a being who was a centre of this whirl of bad forces, they died. And there must have been many of these, a very great number. I saw all that and I understood.

When someone came to see me, I asked to be left alone, I lay quietly in my bed and I passed two or three days absolutely quiet, in concentration, with my consciousness. Subsequently, a friend of ours (a Japanese, a very good friend) came and told me: "Ah! you were ill? So what I thought was true.... Just imagine for the last two or three days, there hasn't been a single new case of illness in the town and most of the people who were ill have been cured and the number of deaths has become almost negligible, and now it is all over. The illness is wholly under control." Then I narrated what had happened to me and he went and narrated it to everybody. They even published articles about it in the papers.

Well, consciousness, to be sure, is more effective than packets of medicine!... The condition was critical. Just imagine, there were entire villages where everyone had died. There was a village in Japan, not very big, but still with more than a hundred people, and it happened, due to an extraordinary chance, that one of the villagers was to receive a letter (the postman went there only if there was a letter; naturally, it was a village far in the countryside); so he went to the countryside;

there was a snowfall; the whole village was under snow... and there was not a living person. It was exactly so. It was that kind of epidemic. And Tokyo was also like that; but Tokyo was a big town and things did not happen in the same fashion. And it was in this way the epidemic ended. That is my story.

Now this brings us naturally to the cure. All that is very well, we now have the knowledge; so, how to prevent illnesses from coming, first of all, and when the illness does occur, how to cure it?

One may try ordinary means and sometimes that succeeds. It is usually when the body is convinced that it has been given the conditions under which it must be all right; it takes the resolution that it must be all right and it is cured. But if your body has not the will, the resolution to get cured, you may try whatever you like, it won't be cured. This also I know by experience. For I knew people who could be cured in five minutes, even of a disease considered very serious, and I knew people who had no fatal illness, but cherished it with such persistence that it did become fatal. It was impossible to persuade their body to let go their illness.

And it is here that one must be very careful and look at oneself with great discrimination to discover the small part in oneself that — how to put it? — takes pleasure in being ill. Oh! there are many reasons. There are people who are ill out of spite, there are people who are ill out of hate, there are people who are ill through despair, there are people... And these are not formidable movements: it is quite a small movement in the being: one is vexed and says: "You will see what is going to happen, you will see the consequences of what he has done to me! Let it come! I am going to be ill." One does not say it openly to oneself, for one would scold oneself, but there is something somewhere that thinks in that way.

So there are two things you have to do when you have discovered the disorder, big or small — the disharmony. Firstly, we said that this disharmony created a kind of tremor and a lack of peace in the physical being, in the body. It is a kind of fever. Even if it is not a fever in general, there is localised fever; there are people who get restless. So the first thing to do is to quieten oneself, bring peace, calm relaxation, with a total confidence, in this little corner (not necessarily in the whole body). Afterwards you see what is the cause of the disorder. You look. Of course, there are many, but still you try to find out approximately the cause of this disorder, and through the pressure of light and knowledge and spiritual force you re-establish the harmony, the proper functioning. And if the ailing part is receptive, if it does not offer any obstinate resistance, you can be cured in a few seconds.

It is not always the case. Sometimes there is, as I have said, a bad will: you are more or less on strike, at least you want the illness to have its consequences. So, that takes a little more time. However, if you do not happen to be particularly ill-willed, after some time the Force acts: after a few minutes or hours or at the most some days you are cured.

Now, in the case of special attacks of adverse forces, the thing gets complicated, because you have not only to deal with the will of the body (note that I do not admit the argument of those who say: "But as for myself I do not want to be ill!", for your consciousness always says that it does not want to be ill, one must be half-crazy to say, "I want to be ill"; but it is not your consciousness that wants to be ill, it is some part of your body or at the most, a fragment of the vital that has gone wrong and wishes to be ill, and unless you observe with a good deal of attention you do not notice it). But I say that the situation gets complicated if behind this there is an attack, a pressure from adverse forces who really want to harm you. You may have opened the door through spiritual error, through a

movement of vanity, of anger, of hatred or of violence; even
if it is merely a movement that comes and goes, that can open
the door. There are always germs watching and only waiting
for an occasion. That is why one should be very careful. Anyhow, for some reason or other, the influence has pierced
through the shell of protection and acts there encouraging the
illness to become as bad as it can be. In that case the first
means is not quite sufficient. Then you have to add something;
you must add the Force of spiritual purification which is such
an absolutely perfectly constructive force that nothing that's
in the least destructive can survive there. If you have this
Force at your disposal or if you can ask for it and get it, you
direct it on the spot and the adverse force usually runs away
immediately, for if it happens to be in the midst of this Force
it gets dissolved, it disappears; for no force of disintegration
can survive within this Force; therefore disintegration disappears and with it that also disappears. It can be changed into
a constructive force, that is possible, or it may be simply dissolved and reduced to nothing. And with that not only is the
illness cured, but all possibility of its return is also eliminated.
You are cured of the illness once and for all, it never comes
back. There you are.

Now, all that is seen on the whole; on the details could
be written books and books. I have given you only general
explanations.

*With the causes you have told us about, one should be
always ill!*

But in ordinary life, most of the time, people are almost always ill — except a few who escape for reasons of a different
order that we shall explain one day. There are very few people who are not more or less ill all the while. But even in or-

dinary life, if within you there is trust, goodwill, a kind of certitude, this kind of inner confidence, oh! as there is in most children perhaps (I do not know, for, after all, those we see here are fairly exceptional), however, there is a trust in life, they are young and they have the feeling that the whole life is before them. Very few things are behind, everything is in front. So that gives them a kind of self-confidence, that pulls them out.

Otherwise, I do not know, in the ordinary life I have known very few people who did not complain of having at least some physical ailment which they carried always with them.... You know perhaps that play of Jules Romain, *Doctor Knock*, in which he says that a healthy man is a sick fellow who is unaware. It is usually true. When you are sufficiently busy not to be all the while occupied with yourself, you do not notice it, but it is there.

22 July 1953

Relation between Body and Mind

When the body falls ill, do the mind and vital also fall ill?

Not necessarily. Illness (I have explained this to you) comes usually from a dislocation between the different parts of the being, from a sort of disharmony. Well, it can very well happen that the body has not followed a certain movement of progress, for instance, that it has remained behind, and that, on the other hand, the other parts of the being have progressed, and so that disequilibrium, that rupture of harmony creates the illness, and the mind may be in a very fine state and the vital also. There are people who have been ill for years — with terrible, incurable diseases — and who have kept their mental capacity marvellously clear and progressed mentally. There is a French poet (a very good poet) called Sully Prudhomme; he was mortally ill; and it was then that he wrote his most beautiful poems. He remained charming, amiable, smiling — amiable with everyone, and yet his body was going to pieces. That depends on people. There are others still — as soon as they feel the least bit ill, everything is upset from top to bottom — they are then good for nothing. For each one the combination is different.

It is said there is a relation between the body and the mind. If the mind is not quite all right, then what?

But certainly there is a relation between the body and the mind! There is even more than a relation: it is a very close tie, for most of the time it is the mind which makes the body ill. In any case, it is the principal factor.

And if the body is not well?

That depends on people, I told you. There are people — as soon as the least thing happens to their body, their mind is completely upset. There are others still who may be very ill and yet keep their mind clear. It is rarer and more difficult to see a mind that's upset and the body remaining healthy — it is not impossible but it is much rarer, for the body depends a great deal on the state of the mind. The mind . . . is the master of the physical being.

23 December 1953

Illnesses Due to Yoga

Can all physical ailments be traced to some disorder in the mind as their ultimate source? If so, what kind of mental disorder would produce such an ailment as, for example, prickly heat or sore throat?

There are as many reasons for an illness as there are people who fall ill; the explanation is different in each case. If you ask me, "Why have I this ailment or that?" I can look and tell you the reason, but there is no general rule.

The ailments of the body are not always the outcome of a mental disorder, disharmony or wrong movement. The source of the malady may be something in the mind, it may be something in the vital; or it may be something more or less purely physical, as in illnesses that arise from an outer contact. Again, the disturbance may be the result of a movement in the Yoga, and in that case too there is a multitude of possible causes.

Let us take up the illnesses that are due to Yoga; for our concern is more directly and intimately with them. Here, although no one reason can be given for any particular illness, yet we can separate them into various groups according to the nature of the causes that provoke them.

The force that comes down into one who is doing Yoga and helps him in his transformation, acts along many different lines and its results vary according to the nature that receives it and the work to be done. First of all, it hastens the transformation of all in the being that is ready to be transformed. If he is open and receptive in his mind, the mind, touched by the power of Yoga, begins to change and progress swiftly. There may be the same rapidity of change in the vital consciousness if that is ready, or even in the body. But in the body the transforming power of Yoga is operative only to a certain degree;

for the receptivity of the body is limited. The most material plane of the universe is still in a condition in which receptivity is mixed with a large amount of resistance. But rapid progress in one part of the being which is not followed by an equivalent progress in other parts produces a disharmony in the nature, a dislocation somewhere; and wherever or whenever this dislocation occurs, it can translate itself into an illness. The nature of the illness depends upon the nature of the dislocation. One kind of disharmony affects the mind and the disturbance it produces may lead even as far as insanity; another kind affects the body and may show itself as fever or prickly heat or any other greater or minor disorder.

On one side, the action of the forces of Yoga hastens the movement of transformation of the being in those parts that are ready to receive and respond to the power that is at work upon it. Yoga, in this way, saves time. The whole world is in a process of progressive transformation; if you take up the discipline of Yoga, you speed up in yourself this process. The work that would require years in the ordinary course, can be done by Yoga in a few days and even in a few hours. But it is your inner consciousness that obeys this accelerating impulse; for the higher parts of your being readily follow the swift and concentrated movement of Yoga and lend themselves more easily to the continuous adjustment and adaptation that it necessitates. The body, on the other hand, is ordinarily dense, inert and apathetic. And if you have in this part something that is not responsive, if there is a resistance here, the reason is that the body is incapable of moving as quickly as the rest of the being. It must take time, it must walk at its own pace as it does in ordinary life. What happens is as when grown-up people walk too fast for children in their company; they have to stop at times and wait till the child who is lagging behind comes up and overtakes them. This divergence between the progress in the inner being and the inertia of the body often creates a dislocation in the system, and that manifests itself as an illness. This is why people who take up Yoga frequently begin by suffering from some physical discomfort or disorder. That need not happen if they are on their guard and careful. Or if there is a greater and unusual receptivity in the body, then too they escape. But an unmixed receptivity making the physical parts closely follow the pace of the inner transformation is hardly possible, unless the body has already been prepared in the past for the processes of Yoga.

In the ordinary life of man a progressive dislocation is the rule. The mental and the vital beings of man follow as best they can the movement of the universal forces, and the stream of the world's inner transformation and evolution carries them a certain way; but the body bound to the law of the most material nature, moves very slowly. After some years, seventy or eighty, a hundred or two hundred, — and that is perhaps the maximum, — the dislocation is so serious that the outer being falls to pieces. The divergence between the demand and the answer, the increasing inability and irresponsiveness of the body, brings about the phenomenon of death. By Yoga the inner transformation that is in slow constant process in the creation is rendered more intense and rapid, but the pace of the outer transformation remains almost the same as in ordinary life. As a result, the disharmony between the inner and the outer being in one who is doing Yoga tends to be all the greater, unless precautions are taken and a protection secured that will help the body to follow the inner march as closely as possible. Even then it is the very nature of the body to hold you back. It is for this reason that to many we are obliged to say, "Do not pull, do not hurry; you must give your body time to follow." Some have to be kept back even for years and not allowed to do much or progress far. Sometimes, to avoid the disequilibrium becomes impossible ; and then you have a disturbance which varies according to the nature of the resistance and the measure of the care you have taken or your negligence. This too is the reason why each time that there is a strong movement of progress, it is almost invariably followed by a period of immobility, which seems to those who are not warned a spell of dullness and stagnation and discouragement in which all progress is stopped, and they think anxiously, "What is the matter? Am I losing time? Nothing is being done." But the truth is that it is the time needed for assimilation; a pause is made for the body to open itself more and become receptive and approach nearer to the level attained by the inner consciousness. The parents have been walking too far ahead; they must halt so that the child left behind may run up and catch them by the hand ; only then can they start again on the journey together.

Each spot of the body is symbolical of an inner movement; there is there a world of subtle correspondences. But this is a long and complex subject and we cannot enter into its details just now. The particular place in the body affected by an illness is an index to the nature of the inner disharmony that has taken place. It points to the origin, it is a sign of the cause of the ailment. It reveals too the nature of the resistance that prevents the whole being from advancing at the same high speed. It indicates the treatment and the cure. If one could perfectly understand where the mistake is, find out what has been unreceptive, open that part and put the force and the light there, it would be possible to re-establish in a moment the harmony that has been disturbed and the illness would immediately go.

The origin of an illness may be in the mind; it may be in the vital; it may be in any of the parts of the being. One and the same illness may be due to a variety of causes; it may spring in different cases from different sources of disharmony. And there may be too an appearance of illness where there is no real illness at all. In that case, if you are sufficiently conscious, you will see that there is just a friction somewhere, some halting in the movement, and by setting it right you will be cured at once. This kind of malady has no truth in it, even when it seems to have physical effects. It is half made up of imagination and has not the same grip on matter as a true illness. . . .

If the whole being could simultaneously advance in its progressive transformation, keeping pace with the inner march of the universe, there would be no illness, there would be no death. But it would have to be literally the whole being integrally from the highest planes, where it is more plastic and yields in the required measure to transforming forces, down to the most material, which is by nature rigid, stationary, refractory to any rapid remoulding change.

There are certain regions which offer a much stronger resistance than others to the action of the Yogic forces, and the illnesses affecting them are harder to cure. They are those parts that belong to the most material layers of the being, and the illnesses that pertain to them, as, for instance, skin diseases or bad teeth. Sri Aurobindo spoke once of a Yogi who, still enjoying robust health and a magnificent physique, had been living for nearly a century on the banks of the Narmada. Offered by a disciple medicine for a toothache, he observed, in refusing, that one tooth had given him trouble for the last two hundred years. This Yogi had secured so much control over material nature as to live two hundred years, but in all that time he had not been able to conquer a toothache.

Some of the diseases which are considered most dangerous are the easiest to cure; some that are considered as of very little importance can offer the most obstinate resistance.

The sources of an illness are manifold and intricate; each can have a multitude of causes, but always it indicates where is the weak part in the being.

16 June 1929

Illness in the Spiritual Life

Sweet Mother, if someone falls seriously ill, is this a purely physical phenomenon or is it a difficulty in his spiritual life?

That depends on the person! If it is someone who is doing yoga, it is quite obviously a difficulty in his spiritual life. If it is somebody who is not at all engaged in yoga and who lives an ordinary life in the most ordinary manner, it is an ordinary accident. It depends absolutely on the person. The outer phenomena may be similar, but the inner causes are absolutely different. No two illnesses are alike, though labels are put on diseases and attempts made to group them; but in fact every person is ill in his own way, and his way depends on what he is, on his state of consciousness and the life he leads.

We have often said that illnesses are always the result of a disturbance of equilibrium, but this disturbance can occur in completely different states of being. For the ordinary man whose consciousness is centred in the physical, outer life, it is a purely physical disturbance of equilibrium, of the functioning of the different organs. But when behind this purely superficial life, an inner life is being fashioned, the causes of illness change; they always become the expression of a disequilibrium between the different parts of the being: between the inner progress or effort and the outer resistances or conditions of one's life, one's body.

Even from the ordinary external point of view, it has been recognised for a very long time that it is a fall in the resistance of the vitality due to immediate moral causes which is always at the origin of an illness. When one is in a normal state of equilibrium and lives in a normal physical harmony, the body has a capacity of resistance, it has within it an atmosphere strong enough to resist illnesses: its most material substance emanates subtle vibrations which have the strength to resist illnesses, even diseases which are called contagious — in fact, all vibrations are contagious, but still, certain diseases are considered as especially contagious. Well, a man who, even from the purely external point of view, is in a state in which his organs function harmoniously and an adequate psychological balance prevails, has at the same time enough resistance for the contagion not to affect him. But if for some reason or other he loses this equilibrium or is weakened by depression, dissatisfaction, moral difficulties or undue fatigue, for instance, this reduces the normal resistance of the body and he is open to the disease. But if we consider someone who is doing yoga, then it is altogether different, in the sense that the causes of disequilibrium are of a different nature and the illness usually becomes the expression of an inner difficulty which has to be overcome.

So each one should find out for himself why he is ill.

19 June 1957

2

MICROBES

Microbes and Yoga

*But are not illnesses sometimes the result of microbes and
not a part of the movement of the Yoga?*

Where does Yoga begin and where does it end? Is not the
whole of your life Yoga? The possibilities of illness are always there in your body and around you; you carry within
you or there swarm about you the microbes and germs of
every disease. How is it that all of a sudden you succumb to
an illness which you did not have for years? You will say it
is due to a "depression of the vital force". But from where
does the depression come? It comes from some disharmony
in the being, from a lack of receptivity to the divine forces.
When you cut yourself off from the energy and light that sustains you, then there is this depression, there is created what
medical science calls a "favourable ground" and something
takes advantage of it. It is doubt, gloominess, lack of confidence, a selfish turning back upon yourself that cuts you off
from the light and divine energy and gives the attack this
advantage. It is this that is the cause of your falling ill and
not microbes.

*But has it not been found that by improved sanitation the
health of the average citizen improves?*

Medicine and sanitation are indispensable in the ordinary
life, but I am not speaking now of the average citizen, I am

speaking of those who do Yoga. Still there is this disadvantage of sanitation that while you diminish the chances of catching an illness, you diminish also your natural power of resistance. Attendants in hospitals, who are always washing with disinfectants, find that their hands become more easily infected and are much more susceptible than the hands of others. There are people, on the contrary, who know nothing of hygiene and do the most insanitary things and yet remain immune. Their very ignorance helps them because it shuts them to the suggestions that come with medical knowledge. On the other hand, your belief in the sanitary precautions you take helps them to work. For your thought is, "Now I am disinfected and safe", and to that extent it makes you safe.

But why then are we to take sanitary precautions such as drinking only filtered water?

Is any one of you pure and strong enough not to be affected by suggestions? If you drink unfiltered water and think, "Now I am drinking impure water", you have every chance of falling sick. And even though such suggestions may not enter through the conscious mind, the whole of your subconscious is there, almost helplessly open to take any kind of suggestion. In life it is the action of the subconscious that has the larger share and it acts a hundred times more powerfully than the conscious parts. The normal human condition is a state filled with apprehensions and fears; if you observe your mind deeply for ten minutes, you will find that for nine out of ten it is full of fears — it carries in it fear about many things, big and small, near and far, seen and unseen, and though you do not usually take conscious notice of it, it is there all the same. To be free from all fear can come only by steady effort and discipline.

And even if by discipline and effort you have liberated your mind and your vital of apprehension and fear, it is more difficult to convince the body. But that too must be done. Once you enter the path of Yoga you must get rid of all fears — the fears of your mind, the fears of your vital, the fears of your body which are lodged in its very cells.

19 May 1929

Moral Conditions: More Important than Physical Ones

Are illnesses tests in the Yoga?

Tests? Not at all.

You are given an illness purposely to make you progress? Surely it is not like that. That is, you may turn the thing round and say that there are people whose aspiration is so constant, whose goodwill so total that whatever happens to them they take as a trial on the path to make progress. I knew people who, whenever they fell ill, took that as a proof of the Divine Grace to help them to progress. They told themselves: it is a good sign, I am going to find out the cause of my illness and I shall make the necessary progress. I knew a few of this kind and they moved on magnificently. There are others, on the contrary, who, far from making use of the thing, let themselves fall flat on the ground. So much the worse for them. But the true attitude when one is ill, is to say: "There is something that is not all right; I am going to see what it is." You must never think that the Divine has purposely sent an illness, for that would truly be a very undesirable Divine!

Even so, there are microbes in water ?

These people are in such a physical, mental, and vital condition that they are liable to catch an illness, even without drinking water, I assure you! Their whole being is a constant disharmony, their whole physical being. I do not mean inwardly, they are perhaps all right there, but those who are all right resist everything.

And I have seen just the contrary. I have seen in this country, here, village people who had only such water as was no longer water to drink, it was mere mud, I have seen it with my own eyes. It was yellowish mud in which cows had bathed and done all the rest and people had waded through it after walking on the roads. They threw their rubbish and everything was in it. And then I saw these people. They entered it, it was, as I said, yellowish mud and there at the end there was a little bit of water — it was not water, it was yellowish, you know — they bent over, collected this water in their palms and drank it. And there were some who did not even allow it to settle. Some knew what to put in it, the herbs needed to make it settle, and if one leaves it sufficiently long it becomes a little clearer. But there were some who knew nothing at all and drank it as it was. And I came to learn that there was just then an epidemic of cholera all around and I said: "There are still people living in that village with that kind of water?" I was told: "We do not have a single case of cholera...." They had become immune, they were habituated. But if there had been a single person who had caught it by chance, probably all would have been dead; for then fear would enter and with fear in them there would be no more resistance, for they were poor miserable things. But it is the moral conditions of these people that are terrible, more than the physical conditions — the moral conditions.

There are sadhus, you know, who accept the conditions of a dirty life through saintliness. They never wash themselves, they have nothing about them that hygiene demands. They live in a truly dirty condition — and they are free from all illness. Probably because they have faith and they do so purposely. Their morale is magnificent.... I am speaking of sincere people and not those who pretend. They have faith. They do not think of their body, they think of the life of their soul. They have no illness. There are some who come to a state in which an arm or a leg or any part of the body has become completely stiff due to their ascetic posture. They cannot move any more; anybody else would die under such conditions; they continue to live because they have faith and they do it purposely, because it is a thing they have imposed on themselves.

Therefore, the moral condition is much more important than the physical. If you were in surroundings where everyone was tidy and then you remained three days without taking a bath, you would fall ill. This is not to say that you should not take a bath! Because we do not want to be sadhus, we want to be yogis. It is not the same thing. And we want the body to take part in the yoga. So we must do whatever is necessary to keep it fit. However, this is only to tell you that the moral condition is much more important than the physical.

Besides, these people, by their asceticism, wilfully spoil their body, torture themselves, yet if it was someone else who did the same thing, people would shout, protest, declare he is a monster. But one does it by one's own choice. And one bears it very well because it is imposed on one's own self and one feels a kind of glory in having done something very "remarkable", through one's aspiration for the divine life!

22 July 1953

What Is a Microbe?

One thing that is now beginning to be recognised by everyone, even by the medical corps, is that hygienic measures, for example, are effective only to the extent that one has confidence in them. Take the case of an epidemic. Many years ago we had a cholera epidemic here — it was bad — but the chief medical officer of the hospital was an energetic man: he decided to vaccinate everybody. When he discharged the vaccinated men, he would tell them, "Now you are vaccinated and nothing will happen to you, but if you were not vaccinated you would be sure to die!" He told them this with great authority. Generally such an epidemic lasts a long time and it is difficult to arrest it, but in some fifteen days, I think, this doctor succeeded in checking it; in any case, it was done miraculously fast. But he knew very well that the best effect of his vaccination was the confidence it gave to people.

Now, quite recently, they have found something else and I consider it wonderful. They have discovered that for every disease there is a microbe that cures it (call it a microbe if you like, anyway, some sort of germ). But what is so extraordinary is that this "microbe" is extremely contagious, even more contagious than the microbe of the disease. And it generally develops under two conditions: in those who have a sort of natural good humour and energy and in those who have a strong will to get well! Suddenly they catch the "microbe" and are cured. And what is wonderful is that if there is one who is cured in an epidemic, three more recover immediately. And this "microbe" is found in all who are cured.

But I am going to tell you something: what people take to be a microbe is simply the materialisation of a vibration or a will from another world. When I learned of these medical discoveries, I said to myself, "Truly, science is making progress." One might almost say with greater reason, "Matter is progressing," it is becoming more and more receptive to a higher will. And what is translated in their science as "microbes" will be perceived, if one goes to the root of things, as simply a vibratory mode; and this vibratory mode is the material translation of a higher will. If you can bring this force or this will, this power, this vibration (call it what you will) into certain given circumstances, not only will it act in you, but also through contagion around you.

14 March 1951

Religious Rules Founded on Hygenic Principles

Almost all superstitions are the result of an experience that is quite local, occasional, exceptional, which has been raised into a mental principle. It is a mental formation, it is not a rule.

Now, there are other instances, as for example a large number of religious rules which are founded solely on hygienic principles, on medical knowledge, and have been raised into religious principles, for that was the only way to make people observe them. If you are not told that "God wants" that you should do this or that, you would not do it, the majority of men ordinarily do not do it. For instance, that very simple thing — washing your hands before eating; in countries where the civilisation is not quite scientific, some people discovered that in truth it was probably more hygienic to wash the hands first! If they had not made a religious rule, if they hadn't said that "God wanted" that a man wash his hands before eating, otherwise it would be an offence against Him, people would have said: "Oh, why? No, not today, tomorrow. I have no time, I am in a hurry!" But in this way there is that constant fear at the back of their minds that something bad will happen to them due to God's anger. This too is a superstition, a big superstition.

15 July 1953

3

FEAR

The Real Disease Is Fear

The real disease is *fear*. Throw the fear away and the disease will go.

*

The first thing from which you must cure once for ever is *Fear*. It is more dangerous than the worst disease.

*

It is the fear — more or less conscious — which does almost all the mischief.

Without fear nothing *can happen.*

*

Do not torment yourself, do not worry; above all try to banish all fear; fear is a dangerous thing which can give importance to something which has none at all. The mere fear of seeing certain symptoms renew themselves is enough to bring about this repetition.

*

My advice is not to worry. More you think of it, more you concentrate upon it and, above all, more you fear, more you give a chance for the thing to grow.

If, on the contrary, you turn your attention and your interest elsewhere you increase the possibilities of cure.

*

All fear must be overcome and replaced by a total confidence in the Divine Grace.

Fear and the Pressure of the Yoga

Nine-tenths of the danger in an illness comes from fear. Fear can give you the apparent symptoms of an illness; and it can give you the illness too, — its effects can go so far as that. Not so long ago the wife of one who frequents the Ashram but is not herself practising Yoga, heard that there was cholera in the house where her milkman lived; fear took her and the next moment she began to show symptoms of the disease. She could however be rapidly cured, because the apparent symptoms were not allowed to develop into the real illness.

There are physical movements, effects of the pressure of the Yoga, which sometimes create ungrounded fears that may do harm if the fear is not rejected. There is, for instance, a certain pressure in the head of which there has been question and which is felt by many, especially in the earlier stages, when something that is still closed has to open. It is a discomfort that comes to nothing and can easily be got over, if you know that it is an effect of the pressure of the forces to which you are opening, when they work strongly on the body to produce a result and to hasten the transformation. Taken quietly, it can turn into a not unpleasurable sensation. But if you get frightened, you are sure to contract a very bad headache; it may even go as far as a fever. The discomfort is due to some resistance in the nature; if you know how to release the resistance, you are immediately free of the discomfort. But get frightened and the discomfort may turn into something much worse. Whatever the character of the experience you have, you must give no room to fear; you must keep an unshaken confidence and feel that whatever happens is the thing that had to happen. Once you have chosen the path, you must boldly accept all the consequences of your choice. But if you choose and then draw back and choose again and again draw back, always wavering, always doubting, always fearful, you create a disharmony in your being, which not only retards your progress, but can be the origin of all kinds of disturbance in the mind and vital being and discomfort and disease in the body.

16 June 1929

Mental, Vital and Physical Fear

Can one get ill through fear?

Yes. I knew someone who was so full of fear that he got cholera! There was cholera in the next house and he got so frightened that he caught the illness and without any other reason, there was no other reason for his catching it: it was through sheer fright. And it is a very common thing; in an epidemic, it is so in the majority of cases. It is through fear that the door is opened and you catch the illness. Those who have no fear can go about freely and generally they catch nothing. But still as I have said there,[1] you may have no fear in the mind, you may have no fear even in the vital, but who has no fear in the body?... Very few.

A strict discipline is needed to cure the body of fear. The cells themselves tremble. It is only by discipline, by yoga that one can overcome this fear. But it is a fact that one can catch anything through fear, even invite an accident. And, you see, from a certain point of view everything is contagious. I knew

[1] *Questions and Answers* 1929 (May 19).

a person who got a wound through the kind of fear that he felt seeing someone else's wound. He really got it.

What is the difference between mental, vital and physical fear?

If you are conscious of the movement of your mind, the movement of your vital and the movement of your physical, you know it.

The mental is very simple: it is thoughts. You begin thinking, for example, there is this illness and this illness is very contagious, perhaps you are going to catch it, and if you catch it, it is going to be a terrible affair and what is to be done so as not to catch it?... So the mind begins to tremble: what is going to happen tomorrow? etc.

The vital, you feel it. You feel it in your sensations. All at once you feel hot, you feel cold, you perspire or all kinds of unpleasant things happen. And then you feel your heart beating fast and suddenly you have fever and then the circulation stops and you become cold.

Physically, well... When you do not any longer have the other two fears, you can become aware of the physical fear. Generally, the other two are much more conscious. They hide the physical fear from you. But when you have no longer any mental or vital fear, then you become aware of it. It is a curious little vibration that gets into your cells and they begin shivering that way. But the cells are not like a heart beating very fast. It is in the very cells: they tremble with just a slight quivering. And it is very difficult to control this. Yet it can be controlled.

I am sure that most of you have felt this as, for example, when one does an exercise which is not done often or does it for the first time; these are tiny little vibrations which seize you in all the cells. And then naturally, you lose your full con-

trol over the movement. The body does not answer to the
Force any more. When you want to put your will to do something, that brings about a kind of resistance and incapacity
in the body. Only, you are not aware of it usually because
your attention is drawn more to the mental apprehension or to
the kind of vital recoil which is very apparent in the consciousness, whereas you are not so very conscious of the resistance
produced in the body. Generally in all sports (athletics and all
competitions), a certain incident occurs: you must have noticed with your friends that some do much better than usual,
while others who usually do well are almost incapacitated at
that moment. They do much worse. Well, this depends on
those small vibrations. Because you lose your full control.
Your will has no longer the full control over the body, for it
vibrates and answers to forces other than yours.... Naturally
I am not speaking of those whose head is in a whirl or whose
vital is altogether upset. Nothing can be done with these, it
is better that they don't try. But I mean those who have
some control over themselves, who undergo the training, to
be sure, but at the time of the competition, cannot do as well
as usual; it depends on a lack of receptivity in the body which
gets this little tremor in the cells of which you are not conscious but which acts as an obstruction. That prevents it from
receiving the Force fully.

22 July 1953

Physical Fear, a Fear in the Cells

From the ordinary point of view, in most cases, it [the cause
of illness] is usually fear — fear, which may be mental fear,
vital fear, but which is almost always physical fear, a fear in
the cells — it is fear which opens the door to all contagion.

Mental fear — all who have a little control over themselves or any human dignity can eliminate it; vital fear is more subtle and asks for a greater control; as for physical fear, a veritable yoga is necessary to overcome it, for the cells of the body are afraid of everything that is unpleasant, painful, and as soon as there is any unease, even if it is insignificant, the cells of the body become anxious, they don't like to be uncomfortable. And then, to overcome that, the control of a conscious will is necessary. It is usually this kind of fear that opens the door to illnesses. And I am not speaking of the first two types of fear which, as I said, any human being who wants to be human in the noblest sense of the word, must overcome, for that is cowardice. But physical fear is more difficult to overcome; without it even the most violent attacks could be repelled. If one has a minimum of control over the body, one can lessen its effects, but that is not immunity. It is this kind of trembling of material, physical fear in the cells of the body which aggravates all illnesses.

Some people are spontaneously free from fear even in their body; they have a sufficient vital equilibrium in them not to be afraid, not to fear, and a natural harmony in the rhythm of their physical life which enables them to reduce the illness spontaneously to a minimum. There are others, on the other hand, with whom the thing always becomes as bad as it can be, sometimes to the point of catastrophe. There is the whole range and this can be seen quite easily. Well, this depends on a kind of happy rhythm of the movement of life in them, which is either harmonious enough to resist external attacks of illness or else doesn't exist or is not sufficiently powerful, and is replaced by that trembling of fear, that kind of instinctive anguish which transforms the least unpleasant contact into something painful and harmful. There is the whole range, from someone who can go through the worst contagion and

epidemics without ever catching anything to one who falls ill
at the slightest chance. So naturally it always depends on the
constitution of each person; and as soon as one wants to make
an effort for progress, it naturally depends on the control one
has acquired over oneself, until the moment when the body
becomes the docile instrument of the higher Will and one can
obtain from it a normal resistance to all attacks.

But when one can eliminate fear, one is almost in safety.
For example, epidemics, or so-called epidemics, like those
which are raging at present — ninety-nine times out of a
hundred they come from fear: a fear, then, which even
becomes a mental fear in its most sordid form, promoted by
newspaper articles, useless talk and so on.

19 June 1957

Why Does One Feel Afraid?

*Why is it so difficult to convince the body [to be free from
fear], when one has succeeded in liberating oneself mentally and vitally?*

Because in the large majority of men, the body receives its
inspirations from the subconscient, it is under the influence of
the subconscient. All the fears driven out from the active
consciousness go and take refuge there and then, naturally,
they have to be chased out from the subconscient and uprooted
from there.

Why does one feel afraid?

I suppose it is because one is egoistic.
There are three reasons. First, an excessive concern about

one's security. Next, what one does not know always gives an uneasy feeling which is translated in the consciousness by fear. And above all, one doesn't have the habit of a spontaneous trust in the Divine. If you look into things sufficiently deeply, this is the true reason. There are people who do not even know that That exists, but one could tell them in other words, "You have no faith in your destiny" or "You know nothing about Grace" — anything whatever, you may put it as you like, but the root of the matter is a lack of trust. If one always had the feeling that it is the best that happens in all circumstances, one would not be afraid.

14 March 1951

The Subconscient Fear of the Body

You must not fear. Most of your troubles come from fear. In fact, ninety percent of illnesses are the result of the subconscient fear in the body. In the ordinary consciousness of the body there is a more or less hidden anxiety about the consequences of the slightest physical disturbance. It can be translated by these words of doubt about the future: "And what will happen?" It is this anxiety that must be checked. Indeed this anxiety is a lack of confidence in the Divine's Grace, the unmistakable sign that the consecration is not complete and perfect.

As a practical means of overcoming this subconscient fear each time that something of it comes at the surface, the more enlightened part of the being must impress on the body the necessity of an entire trust in the Divine's Grace, the certitude that this Grace is always working for the best in ourself as well as in all, and the determination to submit entirely and unreservedly to the Divine's Will.

The body must know and be convinced that its essence is divine and that if no obstacle is put in the way of the Divine's working, nothing can harm us. This process must be steadily repeated until all recurrence of fear is stopped. And then even if the illness succeeds in making its appearance, its strength and duration will be considerably diminished until it is definitively conquered.

14 October 1945

4

ACCIDENTS

Physical Mishaps Come to Teach Equality

Physical mishaps always come as lessons to teach *equality*
and to reveal in us all that is sufficiently pure and luminous to
remain unaffected.

It is in equality that one finds the remedy.

An important point: equality does not mean indifference.

*

*I have been having various kinds of small accidents and
hurts and I feel troubled because all my efforts to avoid
them seem to go in vain. What should I do?*

You need not torture yourself about these small things —
they have no importance in themselves and their utility is to
show us where inconscience is still to be found in our nature
so that we may put light there.

Accidents: Natural Consequences of an Error

*Are illnesses and accidents the results of bad actions or
thoughts, of a fall in one's consciousness? If an error or
a fault which one has committed is the cause, how is one
to know?*

It has nothing to do with *punishment*. They are natural and
normal consequences of an error, of a lack or a fault which

necessarily produces consequences. In fact, in the world everything is a question of equilibrium or disequilibrium, of harmony or disorder. The vibrations of harmony attract and encourage harmonious events; vibrations of disequilibrium create, as it were, disequilibrium in circumstances (illnesses, accidents, etc.). This can be on the collective or on the individual level. But the principle is the same — and so is the remedy: to cultivate in oneself order and harmony, peace and equilibrium, by surrendering to the Divine Will without reserve.

7 July 1965

Accidents: Pessimism and Fear

And when the body has been deformed by illness?

That may be an accident, you know. Accidents are due to many things; in fact they are the result of a conflict of the forces in Nature, a conflict between the forces of growth and progress and the forces of destruction. When there is an accident, an accident that has lasting results, it is always the result of a more or less partial victory of the adverse forces, that is, of the forces of disintegration, disorganisation. That is to be seen.

There are teachings, like that of theosophy for instance, which take Karma in an altogether superficial and human sense and tell you: "Oh! you have met with this accident because in a former life you did something bad, so that comes back upon you in the form of an accident." This is not true, not at all true. This is but human justice, it is neither the justice of Nature nor the justice of the Divine.

Naturally the formation of the body is very important in

this sense that if, for instance, one is constantly under the influence of a depression, of pessimism, discouragement, a lack of faith and trust in life, all this enters, so to say, into one's substance, and then some people, when there is the possibility of an accident, never miss it. Every time there is a chance of something happening to them, they catch it, be it an illness or an accident. You have a whole field of observation here — it is always the same people who meet with accidents. Others do the same things, have as many chances of having an accident, but they are not touched. If you observe their character you will see that the former have a tendency to pessimism and more or less expect something unpleasant to happen to them — and it happens. Or else they are afraid. We know that fear always brings what one fears. If you fear an accident, this acts like a magnet drawing the accident towards you. In this sense, it may be said that it is the result of character. And the same thing holds for illness. There are people who can move about among the sick and in places where there are epidemics and never catch a disease. There are others — it is enough for them to spend an hour with a sick person, they catch the illness. That too depends on what they are within themselves.

And for children, is it also the same thing?

One cannot say. It is a moral question. The problem should not be judged from a moral point of view, one should not say that those who always enjoy good health and to whom nothing happens are "good children" and those who meet with accidents and suffer catastrophes are "bad". That is not correct. For, as I was saying, the logic of Nature is not human logic and its sense of justice (if it has any) is not a human sense. For it there is very little of what we call good and bad.

It could rather be said that there is what is constructive and what is destructive, what is progressive and what is retrogressive. That indeed is very important. And then there are those who are luminous, sunny, happy, smiling and those who are gloomy, dull, misanthropic, dissatisfied, who live in grey shadows. It is the latter who catch all the unpleasant things. Those who are radiant (they may be radiant without it being a spiritual radiance, it may be just a radiation of good sense, balance, an inner confidence, the joy of living), those who carry in themselves the joy of living, these are in harmony with Nature and, being in harmony with Nature, generally avoid accidents, they are immune from diseases and their life develops pleasantly as far as it is possible in the world as it is.

27 January 1954

Accidents: A Slackening of Consciousness

What are the causes of accidents? Are they due to a disequilibrium?

If one answers deeply... Outwardly there are many causes, but there is a deeper cause which is always there. I said the other day that if the nervous envelope is intact, accidents can be avoided, and even if there is an accident it won't have any consequences. As soon as there is a scratch or a defect in the nervous envelope of the being and according to the nature of this scratch, if one may say so, its place, its character, there will be an accident which will correspond to the diminution of resistance in the envelope. I believe almost everybody is psychologically aware of one thing: that accidents occur when one has a sort of uncomfortable feeling, when one is not fully conscious and self-possessed, when one feels uneasy. In any case, generally, people have a feeling that they are not fully themselves, not fully aware of what they are doing. If one were fully conscious, the consciousness wide awake, accidents would not occur; one would make just the right gesture, the necessary movement to avoid the accident. Hence, in an almost absolute way, it is a flagging of consciousness. Or quite possibly it may be that the consciousness is fixed in a higher domain; for example, not to speak of spiritual things, a man who is busy solving a mental problem and is very concentrated upon his mental problem, becomes inattentive to physical things, and if he happens to be in a street or in a crowd, his attention fixed upon his problem, he will not make the movement necessary to avoid the accident, and the accident will occur. It is the same for sports, for games; you can observe this easily, there is always a flagging of the consciousness when accidents occur, or a lack of attention, a little absent-mindedness; suddenly one thinks of something else, the attention is drawn elsewhere — one is not fully conscious of what one is doing and the accident happens.

As I was telling you at the beginning, if for some reason or other — for example, lack of sleep, lack of rest or an absorbing preoccupation or all sorts of things which tire you, that is to say, when you are not above them — if the vital envelope is a little damaged, it does not function perfectly and any current of force whatever which passes through is enough to produce an accident. In the final analysis, the accident comes always from that, it is what one may call inattentiveness or a slackening of consciousness. There are days when one feels quite... not exactly uneasy, but as though one were trying to catch something which escapes, one can't hold together, one is as though half-diluted; these are the days of accidents. You must be attentive. Naturally, this is not to tell you to shut yourself up in your room and not to stir out when you feel like that! This is not what I mean. Rather I mean that you must watch all the more attentively, be all the more on your guard, not allow, precisely, this inattentiveness, this slackening of consciousness to come in.

2 April 1951

5

ADVERSE FORCES

Adverse Forces and the Divine Protection

"What are physical ailments? Are they attacks from hostile forces from outside?"

"There are two factors that have to be considered in the matter. There is what comes from outside and there is what comes from your inner condition. Your inner condition becomes a cause of illness when there is a resistance or revolt in it or when there is some part in you that does not respond to the protection; or even there may be something there that almost willingly and wilfully calls in the adverse forces. It is enough if there is a slight movement of this kind in you; the hostile forces are at once upon you and their attack takes often the form of illness."

The Mother, Questions and Answers 1920

"Some part in you that does not respond to the protection." What does this mean, Mother?

I have already explained it to you. What is it that you do not understand?

I have understood the sense of the words, but I do not understand why it is so.

Because I said "some part of the being"? You understand very well, don't you, what "being under the protection" means? You understand also "going out of the protection"? If you do something contrary, for example, if you are under the protection of the Divine and for a moment you have a thought of doubt or ill-will or revolt, immediately you go out of the protection. So the protection acts around you to prevent adverse forces from coming upon you or an accident from happening, that is to say, even if you lose consciousness, because of the protection even your lack of consciousness will not produce a bad result immediately. But if you go out of the protection and are not all the time vigilant, then either you will be attacked by the adverse forces or an accident will happen.

But those who are not conscious?

Those who are not conscious? But there, too, I have said that I was not speaking of ordinary people. I am not speaking of ordinary people, they are not under a special protection. Ordinary people are under ordinary conditions. They have no special protection watching over them. I am not saying all this for them. They follow all the ordinary laws of life and you cannot explain things to them in the same way.... You were thinking of everybody, that it was so for everybody? It is only for people who do yoga, it is not for everybody.

22 July 1953

Are Mentally Deranged Persons Possessed?

Are mentally deranged people possessed?

Yes, unless there is a physical lesion, a defect in the formation or an accident, a congestion. In all other cases it is always a possession. The proof of it is that if a person is brought to you who is altogether mentally deranged, if he has a lesion, he cannot be cured, while if there is no physical lesion, if it is a possession, then one can cure him. Unfortunately these things happen only to people who like them; there must be in the being much ambition, vanity, combined with much stupidity and a terrible pride — it is on such things that those beings play. I have known cases like that, of persons who were partially possessed, and I succeeded in freeing them from the beings who possessed them. Naturally they felt some relief, a kind of ease for a time, but it did not last long; almost immediately it wore off and they thought: "Now I have become quite an ordinary creature, whereas before I was an exceptional being!" They used to feel within them an exceptional power, even if it was a power to do evil, and they were satisfied with it. So what did they do? They called back with all their force the power they had lost! Of course, the being that had been destroyed could not come back, but as these beings exist in thousands it was replaced by another. I have seen this happen three times consecutively in a case, so much so that in the end I had to tell the person: "I am tired, get rid of it yourself, I am no longer interested!"

8 March 1951

Part II

CURES OF ILLNESS

THE DIVINE GRACE

Universal Nature and the Divine Grace

Justice is the strict logical determinism of the movement of Universal Nature.

Illnesses are this determinism applied to the material body. The medical mind, basing itself upon this ineluctable justice, strives to bring about conditions that should lead logically to good health. . . .

The Divine Grace alone has the power to intervene and change the course of Universal Justice.

The So-called Laws of Nature

I could perhaps add a practical word . . . about the so-called laws of Nature, causes and effects, "inevitable" consequences in the material field, and more particularly from the point of view of health; for example, that if one doesn't take certain precautions, if one doesn't eat as one should, doesn't follow certain rules, necessarily there are consequences.

It is true. But if this is seen in the light of what I have just said, that no two universal combinations are alike, how can laws be established and what is the absolute truth of these laws?... It does not exist.

For, if you are logical, of course with a little higher logic, since no two things, two combinations, two universal manifestations are ever the same, how can anything repeat itself? It can only be an appearance but is not a fact. And to fix rigid laws in this way — not that you cut yourself off from the apparent surface laws, for the mind makes many laws, and the surface very obligingly seems to comply with these laws, but it is only an appearance — but anyway this cuts you off from the creative Power of the Spirit, it cuts you off from the true Power of the Grace, for you can understand that if by your aspiration or your attitude you introduce a higher element, a new element — what we may now call a supramental element — into the existing combinations, you can suddenly change their nature, and all these so-called necessary and ineluctable laws become absurdities. That is to say that you yourself, with your conception, with your attitude and your acceptance of certain alleged principles, you yourself close the door upon the possibility of the miracle — they are not miracles when one knows how they happen, but obviously for the outer consciousness they seem miraculous. And it is you *yourself*, saying to yourself with a logic that seems quite reasonable, "Well, if I do this, that will necessarily happen, or if I don't do that, necessarily this other thing will happen", it is you yourself who close the door — it is as though you were putting an iron curtain between yourself and the free action of the Grace.

How nice it would be to imagine that the Supreme Consciousness, essentially free, presiding at the universal Manifestation, could be full of fantasy in its choice and make things follow one another not according to a logic accessible to human thought but in accordance with another kind of logic, that of the unforeseen!

Then there would no longer be any limits to the possibilities, to the unexpected, the marvellous; and one could hope for the most splendid, the most delightful things from this sovereignly free Will, playing eternally with all the elements and creating unceasingly a new world which logically would have absolutely nothing to do with the preceding one.

Don't you think it would be charming? We have had enough of the world as it is! Why not let it become at least what we think it ought to be?

And I am telling you all this in order that each one of you may put as few barriers as you can in the way of the possibilities to come. That's my conclusion.

I don't know if I have made myself understood, but indeed a day will come, I suppose, when you will know what I meant. That's all, then.

3 October 1956

One Can Modify Destiny

By yogic discipline one can not only foresee destiny but modify it and change it almost totally. First of all, Yoga teaches us that we are not a single being, a simple entity which necessarily has a single destiny that is simple and logical. Rather we have to acknowledge that the destiny of most men is complex, often to the point of incoherence. Is it not this very complexity which gives us the impression of unexpectedness, of indeterminacy and consequently of unpredictability?

To solve the problem one must know that, to begin with, all living creatures, and more especially human beings, are made up of a combination of several entities that come together, interpenetrate, sometimes organising themselves and completing each other, sometimes opposing and contradicting one another. Each one of these beings or states of being belongs to a world of its own and carries within it its own destiny, its own determinism. And it is the combination of all these determinisms, which is sometimes very heterogeneous, that results in the destiny of the individual. But as the organisation and relationship of all these entities can be altered by

personal discipline and effort of will, as these various determinisms act on each other in different ways according to the
concentration of the consciousness, their combination is nearly
always variable and therefore unforeseeable.

For example, the physical or material destiny of a being
comes from his paternal and maternal forebears, from the physical conditions and circumstances in which he is born; one
should be able to foresee the events of his physical life, his
state of health and approximately how long his body will last.
But then there comes into play the formation of his vital being
(the being of desires and passions, but also of impulsive energy
and active will) which brings with it its own destiny. This
destiny affects the physical destiny and can alter it completely
and often even change it for the worse. For example, if a man
born with a very good physical balance, who ought to live in
very good health, is driven by his vital to all kinds of excesses,
bad habits and even vices, he can in this way partly destroy
his good physical destiny and lose the harmony of health and
strength which would have been his but for this unfortunate
interference. This is only one example. But the problem is
much more complex, for, to the physical and vital destinies,
there must be added the mental destiny, the psychic destiny,
and many others besides.

In fact, the higher a being stands on the human scale, the
more complex is his being, the more numerous are his destinies and the more unforeseeable his fate seems to be as a
consequence. This is however only an appearance. The knowledge of these various states of being and their corresponding
inner worlds gives at the same time the capacity to discern the
various destinies, their interpenetration and their combined
or dominant action. Higher destinies are quite obviously the
closest to the central truth of the universe, and if they are allowed to intervene, their action is necessarily beneficent. The

art of living would then consist in maintaining oneself in one's highest state of consciousness and thus allowing one's highest destiny to dominate the others in life and action. So one can say without any fear of making a mistake: be always at the summit of your consciousness and the best will always happen to you. But that is a maximum which is not easy to reach. If this ideal condition turns out to be unrealisable, the individual can at least, when he is confronted by a danger or a critical situation, call upon his highest destiny by aspiration, prayer and trustful surrender to the divine will. Then, in proportion to the sincerity of his call, this higher destiny intervenes favourably in the normal destiny of the being and changes the course of events in so far as they concern him personally. It is events of this kind that appear to the outer consciousness as miracles, as divine interventions.

February 1950

Attitude and the Effect of Things

There is a state in which one realises that the effect of things, circumstances, all the movements and actions of life on the consciousness depends almost exclusively upon one's attitude to these things. There is a moment when one becomes sufficiently conscious to realise that things in themselves are truly neither good nor bad: they are this only in relation to us; their effect on us depends absolutely upon the attitude we have towards them. The same thing, identically the same, if we take it as a gift of God, as a divine grace, as the result of the full Harmony, helps us to become more conscious, stronger, more true, while if we take it — exactly the very same circumstance — as a blow from fate, as a bad force wanting to affect us, this constricts us, weighs us down and takes away from us all con-

sciousness and strength and harmony. And the circumstance
in itself is *exactly* the same — of this, I should like you all to
have the experience, for when you have it, you become master
of yourself. Not only master of yourself but, in what con-
cerns you, master of the circumstances of your life. And this
depends exclusively upon the attitude you take; it is not an
experience that occurs in the head, though it begins there, but
an experience which can occur in the body itself. So much
so, that — well, it is a realisation which naturally asks for a
lot of work, concentration, self-mastery, consciousness pushed
into Matter, but as a result, in accordance with the way the
body receives shocks from outside, the effect may be different.
And if you attain perfection in that field, you become master
of accidents. I hope this will happen. It is possible. It is not
only possible, it is *certain*. Only it is just one step forward.
That is, this power you have — already fully and formidably
realised in the mind — to act upon circumstances to the extent
of changing them totally in their action upon you, that power
can descend into Matter, into the physical substance itself, the
cells of the body, and give the same power to the body in
relation to the things around it.

This is not a faith, it is a certitude that comes from experience.

The experience is not total, but it is there.

This opens new horizons to you; it is the path, it is one step
on the path leading to transformation.

And the logical conclusion is that there is nothing impossible. It is *we* who put limitations. All the time we say, "That
thing is possible, that other, impossible; this, yes, this can be
done, but that, that is impossible." It is *we* who all the time
put ourselves like slaves into the prison of our limits, of our
stupid, narrow, ignorant sense which knows nothing of the
laws of life. The laws of life are not *at all* what you think they

are nor what the most intelligent people think. They are quite different. Taking a step, especially the first step on the path — one begins to find out.

5 May 1954

People Do Not Want the Divine Grace

All the materialism and positivism in the world have been constructed just because people do not want the divine Grace to come in at all. If they are cured they want to say, "It is *I* who cured myself", if they make a progress, they want to think, "It is I who have progressed", if they organise something, they want to proclaim, "It is I who am organising." And many, many of those who try to do otherwise, if they look within themselves, . . . *know* that it is not they who have done the thing, but the divine force.

5 April 1951

2

FAITH

Finally It Is Faith That Cures

We are at a moment of transition in the history of the earth. It is merely a moment in eternal time. But this moment is long compared to human life. Matter is changing to prepare itself for a new manifestation; but the human body is not plastic enough and offers resistance; this is the reason why illnesses and even incomprehensible illnesses are increasing in number and pose a problem for the medical science.

The remedy is in union with the Divine Forces that are at work and a receptivity full of trust and peace that will make the labour easy.

*

Let your receptivity increase this year, to the extent of giving you the power to fully utilise the force that is at work for restoring perfect good health in you.

*

To keep quiet and to concentrate, leaving the Force from above to do its work is the surest way to be cured of anything and everything. There is no illness that can resist that if it is done properly, in time and long enough, with a steady faith and a calm will.

*

You must not lose patience, this does not hasten the cure. You must on the contrary keep a peaceful trust in the fact that you will be cured.

*

My dear child, now it is time for the faith to become truly active and to stand unshaken against all contradictions. Have the faith, the true faith, that you are cured and the cure is bound to come.

*

Finally it is Faith that cures.

*

Physical ailments are always the sign of a resistance in the physical being; but with surrender to the Divine's Will and a complete trust in the working of the Grace, they are bound to disappear soon.

*

It is in proportion to our trust in the Divine that the Divine Grace can act for us and help.

*

We must learn to rely only on the Divine Grace and to call for its help in all circumstances; then it will work out constant miracles.

*

Do not think you are invalid for ever, because the Grace of the Lord is infinite.

A Mental Resolution Is Not Enough

Mother, by a mental effort — for instance, the resolution not to take medicines when one is ill — can one succeed in making the body understand?

That is not enough. A mental resolution is not enough, no. There are subtle reactions in your body which do not obey the mental resolution, it is not enough. Something else is needed.

Other regions must be contacted. A power higher than the mind's is needed. . . .

Mentally, one arrives at very few results, and they are always mixed. Something else is needed. One must pass from the mind into the domain of faith or of a higher consciousness, to be able to act with safety.

It is quite obvious that one of the most powerful means for acting on the body is faith. People who have a simple heart, not a very complicated mind — simple people, you see — who don't have a very great, very complicated mental development but have a very deep faith, have a great power of action over their bodies, very great. That is why one is quite surprised at times: "Here's a man with a great realisation, an exceptional person, and he is a slave of all the smallest physical things, while this man, well, he is so simple and looks so uncouth, but he has a great faith and goes through difficulties and obstacles like a conqueror!"

I don't say that a highly cultured man can't have faith, but it is more difficult, for there is always this mental element which contradicts, discusses, tries to understand, which is difficult to convince, which wants proofs. His faith is less pure. It is necessary, then, to pass on to a higher degree in the evolutionary spiral, pass from the mental to the spiritual; then, naturally, faith takes on a quality of a very high order. But I mean that in daily life, ordinary life, a very simple man who has a very ardent faith can have a mastery over his body — without it being truly a "mastery"; it is simply a spontaneous movement — a control over his body far greater than somebody who has reached a much higher development.

19 June 1957

Dynamic Faith and Absolute Trust

A dynamic faith and a great trust, aren't they the same thing ?

Not necessarily. One should know of what stuff the faith and the trust are made. Because, for instance, if you live normally, under quite normal conditions — without having extravagant ideas and a depressing education — well, through all your youth and usually till you are about thirty, you have an absolute trust in life. If, for example, you are not surrounded by people who, as soon as you have a cold in your head, get into a flurry and rush to the doctor and give you medicines, if you are in normal surroundings and happen to have something — an accident or a slight illness — there is this certainty in the body, this absolute trust that it will be all right: "It is nothing, it will pass off. It is sure to go. I shall be quite well tomorrow or in a few days. It will surely be cured" — whatever you may have caught. That is indeed the normal condition of the body. An absolute trust that all life lies before it and that all will be well. And this helps enormously. One gets cured nine times out of ten, one gets cured very quickly with this confidence: "It is nothing; what is it after all? Just an accident, it will pass off, it is nothing." And there are people who keep it for a very long time, a very long time, a kind of confidence — nothing can happen to them. And what will happen to them is of no importance at all: all will be well, perforce; they have the whole of life before them. Naturally, if you live in surroundings where there are morbid ideas and people pass their time recounting disastrous and catastrophic things, then you may think wrongly. And if you think wrongly, this reacts on your body. Otherwise, the body as it is can keep this confidence till the age of forty or fifty — it depends upon people

— some know how to live a normal, balanced life. But the body is quite confident about its life. It is only if thought comes in and brings all kinds of morbid and unhealthy imaginations, as I said, that it changes everything. I have seen instances like that: children who had these little accidents one has when running and playing about: they did not even think about it. And it disappeared immediately. I have seen others whose family has drummed into them since the time they could understand, that everything is dangerous, that there are microbes everywhere, that one must be very careful, that the least wound may prove disastrous, that one must be altogether on one's guard and take great care that nothing serious happens.... So, they must have their wounds dressed, must be washed with disinfectants, and there they set wondering: "What is going to happen to me? Oh! I may perhaps get tetanus, a septic fever...." Naturally, in such cases one loses confidence in life and the body feels the effects keenly. Three-fourths of its resistance disappears. But normally, naturally, it is the body which knows that it must remain healthy, and it knows it has the power to react. And if something happens, it tells this something: "It is nothing, it will go away, don't think about it, it is over"; and it does go.

That of course is absolute trust.

Now, you are speaking of "dynamic faith". Dynamic faith is something different. If one has within him faith in the divine grace, that the divine grace is watching over him, and that no matter what happens the divine grace is there, watching over him, this one may keep all one's life and always; and with this one can pass through all dangers, face all difficulties, and nothing stirs, for you have the faith and the divine grace is with you. It is an infinitely stronger, more conscious, more lasting force which does not depend upon the conditions of your physical build, does not depend upon anything except the divine grace alone, and hence it leans on the Truth and nothing can shake it. It is very different.

7 October 1953

Will-power and the Divine Power

What should one do who wants to change his bodily condition, effect a cure or correct some physical imperfection? Should he concentrate upon the end to be realised and exercise his will-power or should he only live in the confidence that it will be done or trust in the Divine Power to bring about the desired result in its own time and in its own way?

All these are so many ways of doing the same thing and each in different conditions can be effective. The method by which you will be most successful depends on the consciousness you have developed and the character of the forces you are able to bring into play. You can live in the consciousness of the completed cure or change and by the force of your inner formation slowly bring about the outward change. Or if you know and have the vision of the force that is able to effect these things and if you have the skill to handle it, you can call it down and apply it in the parts where its action is needed, and it will work out the change. Or, again, you can present your difficulty to the Divine and ask of It the cure, putting confidently your trust in the Divine Power.

But whatever you do, whatever the process you use, and even if you happen to have acquired in it a great skill and power, you must leave the result in the hands of the Divine.

Always you may try, but it is for the Divine to give you the
fruit of your effort or not to give it. There your personal
power stops; if the result comes, it is the Divine Power and
not yours that brings it. You question if it is right to ask the
Divine for these things. But there is no more harm in turning to the Divine for the removal of a physical imperfection
than in praying for the removal of a moral defect. But whatever you ask for or whatever your effort, you must feel, even
while trying your best, using knowledge or putting forth
power, that the result depends upon the Divine Grace. Once
you have taken up the Yoga, whatever you do must be done
in a spirit of complete surrender. This must be your attitude, — "I aspire, I try to cure my imperfections, I do my
best, but for the result I put myself entirely into the hands
of the Divine."

> *Does it help, if you say, "I am sure of the result, I know
> that the Divine will give me what I want"?*

You may take it in that way. The very intensity of your
faith may mean that the Divine has already chosen that the
thing it points to shall be done. An unshakable faith is a sign
of the presence of the Divine Will, an evidence of what shall
be.

23 June 1929

Awaken Faith in the Cells of the Body

You must tell a child — or yourself if you are no longer quite
a baby — "Everything in me that seems unreal, impossible,
illusory, *that* is what is true, *that* is what I must cultivate."
When you have these aspirations: "Oh, not to be always

limited by some incapacity, all the time held back by some bad will!", you must cultivate within you this certitude that *that is* what is essentially true and *that is* what must be realised.

Then faith awakens in the cells of the body. And you will see that you find a response in your body itself. The body itself will feel that if its inner will helps, fortifies, directs, leads, well, all its limitations will gradually disappear.

And so, when the first experience comes, which sometimes begins when one is very young, the first contact with the inner joy, the inner beauty, the inner light, the first contact with *that*, which suddenly makes you feel, "Oh! that is what I want," you must cultivate it, never forget it, hold it constantly before you, tell yourself, "I have felt it once, so I can feel it again. This has been real for me, even for the space of a second, and that is what I am going to revive in myself".... And encourage the body to seek it — to seek it, *with the confidence* that it carries that possibility within itself and that if it calls for it, it will come back, it will be realised again.

This is what should be done when one is young. This is what should be done every time one has the opportunity to recollect oneself, commune with oneself, seek oneself.

And then you will see. When one is normal, that is to say, unspoilt by bad teaching and bad example, when one is born and lives in a healthy and relatively balanced and normal environment, the body, spontaneously, without any need for one to intervene mentally or even vitally, has the certitude that even if something goes wrong it will be cured. The body carries within itself the certitude of cure, the certitude that the illness or disorder is sure to disappear. It is only through the false education from the environment that gradually the body is taught that there are incurable diseases, irreparable accidents, and that it can grow old, and all these stories which destroy its faith and trust. But normally, the body of a normal child — the body, I am not speaking of the thought — the body itself feels when something goes wrong that it will certainly be all right again. And if it is not like that, this means that it has already been perverted. It seems *normal* for it to be in good health, it seems quite abnormal to it if something goes wrong and it falls ill; and in its instinct, its spontaneous instinct, it is sure that everything will be all right. It is only the perversion of thought which destroys this; as one grows up the thought becomes more and more distorted, there is the whole collective suggestion, and so, little by little, the body loses its trust in itself, and naturally, losing its self-confidence, it also loses the spontaneous capacity of restoring its equilibrium when this has been disturbed.

But if when very young, from your earliest childhood, you have been taught all sorts of disappointing, depressing things — things that cause decomposition, I could say, disintegration — then this poor body does its best but it has been perverted, put out of order, and no longer has the sense of its inner strength, its inner force, its power to react.

If one takes care not to pervert it, the body carries within itself the certitude of victory. It is only the wrong use we make of thought and its influence on the body which robs it of this certitude of victory. So, the first thing to do is to cultivate this certitude instead of destroying it; and when it is there, no effort is needed to aspire, but simply a flowering, an unfolding of that inner certitude of victory.

The body carries within itself the sense of its divinity. There. This is what you must try to find again in yourself if you have lost it.

When a child tells you a beautiful dream in which he had many powers and all things were very beautiful, be very care-

ful never to tell him, "Oh! life is not like that", for you are
doing something wrong. You must on the contrary tell him,
"Life *ought to be* like that, and *it will be* like that!"

31 July 1957

3

ASPIRATION

Do Not Love Your Ill-health

Do not love your ill-health and the ill-health will leave you.

*

Wake up in your self a will to conquer. Not a mere will in the mind but a will in the very cells of your body. Without that you can't do anything, e.g. you may take a hundred medicines but they won't cure you unless you have a will to overcome the physical illness.

*

As many cases
so many cures
The most important thing in therapeutics is to teach the body to react properly and reject the illness.
   Blessings.

*

The body should reject illness as energetically as in the mind we reject falsehood.

*

The body is cured if it has decided to be cured.

Physical Aspiration

You may have a physical aspiration also; that the body may feel the need to acquire a kind of equipoise in which all the parts of the being will be well balanced, and that you may have the power to hold off illness at a distance or overcome it fast when it enters trickily, and that the body may always function normally, harmoniously, in perfect health. That is a physical aspiration. . . .

How can the physical manage to aspire, since it is the mind that thinks?

As long as it is the mind that thinks, your physical is something that's three-fourths inert and without its own consciousness. There is a physical consciousness proper, a consciousness of the body; the body is conscious of itself, and it has its own aspiration. So long as one thinks of one's body, one is not in one's physical consciousness. The body has a consciousness that's quite personal to it and altogether independent of the mind. The body is completely aware of its own functioning or its own equilibrium or disequilibrium, and it becomes absolutely conscious, in quite a precise way, if there is a disorder somewhere or other, and (how shall I put it?) it is in contact with that and feels it very clearly, even if there are no external symptoms. The body is aware if the whole working is harmonious, well balanced, quite regular, functioning as it should; it has that kind of plenitude, a sense of plenitude, of joy and strength — something like the joy of living, acting, moving in an equilibrium full of life and energy. Or else the body can be aware that it is ill-treated by the vital and the mind and that this harms its own equilibrium, and it suffers from this. That may produce a complete disequilibrium in it. And so on. . . .

And so, when one has developed this body-consciousness, one can have a very clear perception of the opposition between the different kinds of consciousness. When the body needs something and is aware that this is what it needs, and the vital wants something else and the mind yet another, well, there may very well be a discussion among them, and contradictions and conflicts. And one can discern very clearly what the poise of the body is, the need of the body in itself, and in what way the vital interferes and destroys this equilibrium most often and harms the development so much, because it is ignorant. And when the mind comes in, it creates yet another disorder which is added to the one between the vital and the physical, by introducing its ideas and norms, its principles and rules, its laws and all that, and as it doesn't take into account exactly the needs of the other, it wants to do what everybody does. Human beings have a much more delicate and uncertain health than animals because their mind intervenes and disturbs the equilibrium. The body, left to itself, has a very sure instinct. For instance, never will the body if left to itself eat when it doesn't need to or take something which will be harmful to it. And it will sleep when it needs to sleep, it will act when it needs to act. The instinct of the body is very sure. It is the vital and the mind which disturb it: one by its desires and caprices, the other by its principles, dogmas, laws and ideas. And unfortunately, in civilisation as it is understood, with the kind of education given to children, this sure instinct of the body is completely destroyed: it is the rest that dominate. And naturally things happen as they do: one eats things that are harmful, one doesn't take rest when one needs to or sleeps too much when it is not necessary or does things one shouldn't do and spoils one's health completely.

7 October 1953

Spontaneous Aspiration in the Body

You ask how it [aspiration] can be spontaneous? Even in the body, for instance, when there is something like an attack, an accident, an illness trying to come in — something — an attack on the body, a body that is left to its natural spontaneity has an urge, an aspiration, a spontaneous will to call for help. But as soon as the affair goes to the head, it takes the form of things to which one is accustomed: everything is spoilt. But if the body is seen in itself, just as it is, there is something which suddenly wakes up and calls for help, and with such a faith, such an intensity, just as the tiny little baby calls its mamma, you know — or whoever is there, it says nothing if it cannot speak. But the body left to itself without this kind of constant action of the mind upon it... well, it has this: as soon as there is some disturbance, immediately it has an aspiration, a call, an effort to seek help, and this is very powerful. If nothing intervenes, it is very powerful. It is as though the cells themselves sprang up in an aspiration, a call.

In the body there are invaluable and unknown treasures. In all its cells, there is an intensity of life, of aspiration, of the will to progress which one does not usually even realise. The body-consciousness would have to be completely warped by the action of the mind and vital for it not to have an immediate will to re-establish the equilibrium. When this will is not there, it means that the entire body-consciousness has been spoilt by the intervention of the mind and vital. In people who cherish their malady more or less subconsciously with a sort of morbidity under the pretext that it makes them interesting, it is not their body at all — poor body! — it is something they have imposed upon it with a mental or vital perversion. The body, if left to itself, is remarkable, for, not only does it aspire for equilibrium and well-being but it is capable of restoring the balance. If one leaves one's body alone without intervening with all those thoughts, all the vital reactions, all the depressions, and also all the so-called knowledge and mental constructions and fears — if one leaves the body to itself, spontaneously it will do what is necessary to set itself right again.

The body in its natural state likes equilibrium, likes harmony; it is the other parts of the being which spoil everything.

Mother, how can one prevent the mind from intervening?

Ah! first you must will it, and then you must say, as to people who make a lot of noise, "Keep quiet, be quiet, be quiet!"; you must do this when the mind comes along with all its suggestions and all its movements. You must tranquillise it, pacify it, make it silent. The first thing is not to listen to it. Most of the time, as soon as all these come, all these thoughts, one looks, seeks to understand, one listens; then naturally that imbecile believes that you are very much interested: it increases its activity. You must not listen, must not pay attention. If it makes too much noise, you must tell it: "Be still! Now then, silence, keep quiet!" without making a lot of noise yourself, you understand? You must not imitate those people who begin shouting: "Keep quiet", and make such a noise themselves that they are even noisier than the others!

19 May 1954

PEACE

A Great Remedy for Disease

Peace and stillness are the great remedy for disease.
When we can bring peace in our cells we are cured.

*

Catch hold of a peace deep within and push it into the cells of the body. With the peace will come back the health.

*

Establish a greater peace and quietness in your body, that will give you the strength to resist attacks of illness.

*

The imperative condition for cure is calm and quietness. Any agitation, any narrowness prolongs the illness.

*

(Regarding stomach trouble)

It is due to restlessness and agitation. What is the matter? Bring down peace, the *Divine Peace*, in your stomach and it will be all right.

*

I am having fever; what is the best way to get rid of it?

Remain peaceful and confident and it will soon be over.

GOOD FORMATIONS

Get Out of Wrong Thinking

We are always surrounded by the things of which we think.

*

Those who think falsely will live in falsehood and misery. Get out of wrong thinking and you will get out of suffering.

An old wise man in China has written, "Thought creates for itself its own suffering."

*

I feel a darkness obstructing the back of my head. My head feels heavy and dark. Why has this happened to me and what is it?

Most often these attacks are the result of the bad thoughts you have had, which fall back on you.

Be Always Benevolent

One advice given here [in the Dhammapada] is to be always benevolent. You must not take it as an advice of the commonplace type. It says quite an interesting thing, very interesting even: I comment on it, "Be benevolent and you will be free from suffering, be always contented and happy, you will radiate your quiet happiness."

Be always kind, come out of all bitter criticism, see no more evil in everything, obstinately force yourself to see nothing but the kind Presence of the divine Grace and you will see not only within you but around you, an atmosphere of quiet joy, peaceful trust, luminous hope spreading more and more and not only will you feel happy and quiet yourself but the major part of your bodily disorders will disappear.

It is quite remarkable that the digestive functions are extremely sensitive to a critical, unkind, sour attitude, a harsh judgment. Nothing more than that and the functioning of digestion is disturbed. And it is a vicious circle: the more the digestive function is disturbed, the more you become unkind, critical, disgusted with life and things and persons. So you do not come out of it. There is only one cure, namely, to deliberately come out of this attitude, to refuse absolutely to have it and to force on yourself, through constant control, a willed attitude of thorough kindliness. Try and you will see that you are much better in health.

22 August 1958

Happy Formations, Formations of Light

Ah! I wanted to ask you a question. We said at the beginning: one is surrounded by what one thinks about. You understand quite well what this means? (*Turning to a child*) Every time you think of something, it is as though you had a magnet in your hand and were attracting that thing towards yourself — you understand. Now, there are people who have a very, very bad habit of always thinking about all possible catastrophes, and are in a sort of constant apprehension about some calamity befalling them the next moment. I know many like that, there are some here. And so, those people have as though a magnet in their hands to attract calamities, not only upon themselves but upon others also. That lays a big responsibility upon them. And if one can't stop all the time from thinking about something — some have a head that runs on and they haven't found a way of stopping it — well, why not make it run on the right lines instead of letting it run on the others! Once your head begins to run, let it run on all the good things that can happen. If it is obliged to turn round and round, well, turn then to the good side! That is, if somebody is ill, instead of saying: "What is going to happen, perhaps this is going to be very serious, and if it is that disease... and a calamity comes so quickly", instead of all that, if one thinks: "Oh! that is nothing, illnesses are outer illusions translating some deeper vibrations which are not seen, that is why one doesn't speak about them, but that's how it is. And these deeper vibrations may come and set in order what has been disturbed. And this imbalance, this illness or bad thing that has come, well, it will be absorbed by the Grace and will disappear, no trace of it will remain, except that of things agreeable and pleasant." One may continue to think in this way uninterruptedly.... People always need to make their mind run, run, run, but then make it run on the right lines, you will see that it has an effect. For instance, let it go like this: that I shall learn better and better, shall know better and better, become healthier and healthier, and all difficulties will vanish, and wicked people will become sweet and good, and ill people will be cured, and houses which should be built will be built, and those things which should disappear will disappear, but giving place to better things, and the world will move in a constant progress, and at the end of that progress there will be a total harmony, and so on, and continue thus.... You can go on endlessly. But then you will have around you and around your head all kinds of pretty things. Those who perceive the atmosphere see certain inky stains, like an octopus there, yes, like that, with its tentacles to try and upset your mind — instead of that, one will see happy formations, formations of light or rays of sunlight or perhaps beautiful pictures, all that. One will see beautiful things — there are painters who do that and they always catch thoughts.

9 December 1953

Mind: A Considerable Power of Formation

The mind . . . is the master of the physical being. And I have said the latter was a very docile and obedient servant. Only one doesn't know how to use one's mind, rather the opposite. Not only does one not know how to use it, but one uses it ill — as badly as possible. The mind has a considerable power of formation and a direct action on the body, and usually one uses this power to make oneself ill. For as soon as the least thing goes wrong, the mind begins to shape and build all the catastrophes possible, to ask itself whether it could be this, whether it could be that, if it is going to be like that, and how it will all end. Well, if instead of letting the mind do this disastrous work, one used the same capacity to make favourable formations — simply, for example, to give confidence to the body, to tell it that it is just a passing disturbance and that it is nothing, and if it enters a real state of receptivity, the disorder will disappear as easily as it has come, and one can cure oneself in a few seconds — if one knows how to do that, one gets wonderful results.

23 December 1953

Imagination: A Power of Formation

Imagination is a power of formation. In fact, people who have no imagination are not formative from the mental point of view, they cannot give a concrete power to their thought. Imagination is a very powerful means of action. For instance, if you have a pain somewhere and if you imagine that you are making the pain disappear or are removing it or destroying it — all kinds of images like that — well, you succeed perfectly.

There's a story of a person who was losing her hair at a fantastic rate, enough to become bald within a few weeks, and then someone told her, "When you brush your hair, imagine that it is growing and will grow very fast." And always, while brushing her hair, she said, "Oh! my hair is growing, oh! it will grow very fast...." — and it happened! But what people usually do is to tell themselves, "Ah! all my hair is falling again and I shall become bald, that's certain, it's going to happen!"

And of course it happens!

27 August 1958

Mantra: An Extraordinary Effect

When you are playing and suddenly become aware that something is going wrong — you are making mistakes, are inattentive, sometimes opposing currents come across what you are doing — if you develop the habit, automatically at this moment, of calling as by a mantra, of repeating a word, that has an extraordinary effect. You choose your mantra; or rather, one day it comes to you spontaneously in a moment of difficulty. At a time when things are very difficult, when you have a sort of anguish, anxiety, when you don't know what is going to happen, suddenly this springs up in you, the word springs up in you. For each one it may be different. But if you mark this and each time you face a difficulty you repeat it, it becomes irresistible. For instance, if you feel you are about to fall ill, if you feel you are doing badly what you are doing, if you feel something evil is going to attack you, then.... But it must be a spontaneity in the being, it must spring up from you without your needing to think about it: you choose your mantra because it is a spontaneous expression of your aspiration; it may be one word, two or three words, a sentence, that depends on each one, but it must be a sound which awakens in you a certain condition. Then, when you have that, I assure you that you can pass through everything without difficulty. Even in the face of a real, veritable danger, an attack, for instance, by someone who wants to kill you, if, without getting excited, without being perturbed, you quietly repeat your mantra, one can do nothing to you. Naturally, you must truly be master of yourself; one part of the being must not be trembling there like a leaf; no, you must do it entirely, sincerely, then it is all-powerful. The best is when the word comes to you spontaneously: you call in a moment of great difficulty (mental, vital, physical, emotional, whatever it may be) and suddenly that springs up in you, two or three words, like magical words. You must remember these and form the habit of repeating them in moments when difficulties come. If you form the habit, one day it will come to you spontaneously: when the difficulty comes, at the same time the mantra will come. Then you will see that the results are wonderful. But it must not be an artificial thing or something you arbitrarily decide: "I shall use those words"; nor should somebody else tell you, "Oh! you know, this is very good" — it is perhaps very good for him but not for everyone.

5 May 1951

Correct Attitude and Illness

X had an accident in the knee long ago and this leg is a little weaker than the other one, there was just a possibility of an upsetting. She noticed that so long as she had the correct attitude she *felt nothing*, there was nothing, it seemed to have gone altogether. As soon as she fell back into the ordinary consciousness, the illness returned.... And she had had innumerable experiences. I found it very interesting. Others also.

And it is truly interesting. It is truly interesting because it has a clarity altogether limpid and obvious, because it is *solely a state of consciousness.* When one has the consciousness (that is to say, as the consciousness grows more and more true — not something that is arrested, but a consciousness that is ascending), when you are within that, everything is all right: as soon as you fall back into the old unprogressive consciousness or progressing slowly, imperceptibly, then the disorder returns. And that is as though a lesson given in an altogether clear and obvious way.

10 December 1969

6

THE NERVOUS ENVELOPE

The Nervous Envelope Protects the Body

The vital body surrounds the physical body with a kind of envelope which has almost the same density as the vibrations of heat observable when the day is very hot. And it is this which is the intermediary between the subtle body and the most material vital body. It is this which protects the body from all contagion, fatigue, exhaustion and even from accidents. Therefore if this envelope is wholly intact, it protects you from everything, but a little too strong an emotion, a little fatigue, some dissatisfaction or any shock whatsoever is sufficient to scratch it as it were and the slightest scratch allows any kind of intrusion. Medical science also now recognises that if you are in perfect vital equilibrium, you do not catch illness or in any case you have a kind of immunity from contagion. If you have this equilibrium, this inner harmony which keeps the envelope intact, it protects you from everything. There are people who lead quite an ordinary life, who know how to sleep as one should, eat as one should, and their nervous envelope is so intact that they pass through all dangers as though unconcerned. It is a capacity one can cultivate in oneself. If one becomes aware of the weak spot in one's envelope, a few minutes' concentration, a call to the force, an inner peace is sufficient for it to be all right, get cured, and for the untoward thing to vanish.

27 January 1951

The Nervous Envelope: A Perfect Protection

To whatever cause an illness may be due, material or mental, external or internal, it must, before it can affect the physical body, touch another layer of the being that surrounds and protects it. This subtler layer is called in different teachings by various names, — the etheric body, the nervous envelope. It is a subtle body and yet almost visible. In density something like the vibrations that you see around a very hot and steaming object, it emanates from the physical body and closely covers it. All communications with the exterior world are made through this medium, and it is this that must be invaded and penetrated first before the body can be affected. If this envelope is absolutely strong and intact, you can go into places infested with the worst of diseases, even plague and cholera, and remain quite immune. It is a perfect protection against all possible attacks of illness, so long as it is whole and entire, thoroughly consistent in its composition, its elements in faultless balance. This body is built up, on the one side, of a material basis, but rather of material conditions than of physical matter, on the other, of the vibrations of our psychological states. Peace and equanimity and confidence, faith in health, undisturbed repose and cheerfulness and bright gladness constitute this element in it and give it strength and substance. It is a very sensitive medium with facile and quick reactions; it readily takes in all kinds of suggestions and these can rapidly change and almost remould its condition. A bad suggestion acts very strongly upon it; a good suggestion operates in the contrary sense with the same force. Depression and discouragement have a very adverse effect; they cut out holes in it, as it were, in its very stuff, render it weak and unresisting and open to hostile attacks an easy passage.

It is the action of this medium that partly explains why

people often feel a spontaneous and unreasoning attraction or repulsion for each other. The first seat of these reactions is in this protecting envelope. Easily we feel attracted towards people who bring a reinforcement to our nervous envelope; we are repelled by those who disturb or hurt it. Whatever gives it a sense of expansion and comfort and ease, whatever makes it respond with a feeling of happiness and pleasure exercises on us at once an attraction; when the effect is in the contrary sense, it responds with a protecting repulsion. This movement, when two people meet, is often mutual. It is not, of course, the only cause of affinities, but it is one and a very frequent cause.

16 June 1929

Illnesses Enter through the Subtle Body

Illnesses enter through the subtle body, don't they? How can they be stopped?

Ah! here we are.... If one is very sensitive, very sensitive — one must be very sensitive — the moment they touch the subtle body and try to pas through, one feels it. It is not like something touching the body, it is a sort of feeling. If you are able to perceive it at that moment, you have still the power to say "no", and it goes away. But for this one must be extremely sensitive. However, that develops. All these things can be developed methodically by the will. You can become quite conscious of this envelope, and if you develop it sufficiently, you don't even need to look and see, you feel that something has touched you. . . .

. . .One can very easily feel a kind of little discomfort (it is not something which is imposed with a great force), a little

uneasiness coming near you from anywhere at all: front, behind, above, below. If at that moment you are sufficiently
alert, you say "no", as though you were cutting off the contact
with great strength, and it is finished. If you are not conscious at that moment, the next minute or a few minutes later
you get a queer sick feeling inside, a cold in the back, a little
uneasiness, the beginning of some disharmony; you feel a
maladjustment somewhere, as though the general harmony
had been disturbed. Then you must concentrate all the more
and with a great strength of will keep the faith that nothing
can do you harm, nothing can touch you. This suffices, you
can throw off the illness at that moment. But you must do this
immediately, you understand, you must not wait five minutes,
it must be done at once. If you wait too long and begin to feel
really an uneasiness somewhere, and something begins to get
quite disturbed, then it is good to sit down, concentrate and
call the Force, concentrate it on the place which is getting disturbed, that is to say, which is beginning to become ill. But if
you don't do anything at all, an illness indeed gets lodged somewhere; and all this, because you were not sufficiently alert.
And sometimes one is obliged to follow the entire curve to find
the favourable moment again and get rid of the business. I
have said somewhere that in the physical domain all is a question of method — a method is necessary for realising everything. And if the illness has succeeded in touching the
physical-physical, well, you must follow the procedure needed
to get rid of it. This is what medical science calls "the course of
the illness". One can hasten the course with the help of spiritual forces, but all the same the procedure must be followed.
There are some four different stages. The very first is instan-
taneous. The second can be done in some minutes, the third
may take several hours and the fourth several days. And then,
once the thing is lodged there, all will depend not only on the

receptivity of the body but still more on the willingness of the part which is the cause of the disorder. You know, when the thing comes from outside it is in affinity with something inside. If it manages to pass through, to enter without one's being aware of it, it means there is some affinity somewhere, and the part of the being which has responded must be convinced.

I have known some truly extraordinary instances. 'If you can at the moment... Wait, take an example which is quite concrete: sunstroke. This upsets you considerably, it is one of the things which makes you most ill — a sunstroke upsets everything, it disturbs the inner functions, it generally causes a congestion in the head and very high fever. So, if this has happened, if it has succeeded in getting through the protection and entering you, well, if you can just go into a quiet place, stretch yourself out flat, go out of your body (naturally, you must learn this; there are people who do this spontaneously, for others a long discipline is necessary), go out of your body, remain above in a way to be able to see the body (you know the phenomenon, seeing one's body when one is outside? this can be done at will, going out of one's body and remaining just above it), the body is stretched out on a bed, a bench, on the ground, anywhere; you are stretched just above it and from there, consciously, you pull the Force from above, and if you are used to doing it, if your aspiration is strong enough, you get the answer; and then, from there, taking care not to re-enter your body, you begin to push these forces into the body, like that, regularly, until you see the body receiving them (for, the first few moments they don't enter, because the body is quite upset by the illness, it is not receptive, it is curled up), you push them gently, gently, quietly, without nervousness, very peacefully, into the body. But you must not be disturbed by anyone. If someone comes along, sees you stretched out and shakes you, it is extremely dangerous. You must do this in quiet conditions, ask people not to disturb you or better shut yourself up where they can't disturb you. But you can concentrate slowly (this takes more or less time — ten minutes, half an hour, one hour, two hours — it depends upon the seriousness of the disorder which has set in), slowly, from above, you concentrate the Force until you see that the body is receiving, that the Force is entering, the disorder is being set right and there is a relaxation in the body itself. Once that is done you can get back and you are cured. This has been done for a sunstroke, which is a fairly violent thing, and also for typhoid fever, and many other illnesses, as, for instance, for a liver which was suddenly upset somehow (not due to indigestion, but a liver which doesn't function properly for the moment); it may also be cured in the same way. There was a case of cholera which was healed like that. The cholera had just been caught, had entered, but was not yet lodged; it was completely cured. Consequently, when I say that if one masters the spiritual force and knows how to use it, there is no malady which cannot be cured, I don't say it just like that in the air; it is said from experience with the thing. Of course, you will say you don't know how to go out of the body, draw the Force, concentrate it, have all this mastery.... It is not very frequent, but it is not impossible. And one can be sure that if one is helped... In fact, there is a much easier method, it is to call for help.

But the condition in every case — in every case — whether one does it oneself and depending only on oneself or whether one does it by asking someone to do it for one, the first condition: not to fear and to be calm. If you begin to boil and get fidgety in your body, it is finished, you can do nothing.

For everything — to live the spiritual life, heal sickness — for everything, one must be calm.

31 March 1951

7

ACCIDENTS

Accidents and an Awakened Consciousness

There is a moment for choice, even in an accident. For instance, one slips and falls. Just between the moment one has slipped and the moment one falls there is a fraction of a second. At that moment one has the choice: it may be nothing much, it may be very serious. Only, the consciousness must naturally be wide awake and one must be in contact with one's psychic being constantly — there is no time to make the contact, one must *be* in contact. Between the moment one slips and the moment one is on the ground, if the mental and psychic formation is sufficiently strong, then there is nothing, nothing will happen — nothing happens. But if at that moment, the mind according to its habit becomes a pessimist and tells itself: "Ai! I have slipped...." That lasts the fraction of a second; that doesn't take even a minute, it is a fraction of a second; during a fraction of a second one has the choice. But one must be so awake, every minute of one's life! For a fraction of a second one has the choice, there is a fraction of a second in which one can prevent the accident from being serious, can prevent the illness from entering in. One always has the choice. But it is for a fraction of a second and one must not miss it. If one misses it, it is finished.

One can make it afterwards? (Laughter)

No. Afterwards there is yet another moment.... One has fallen, one is already hurt; but there is still a moment when one can change things for the better or worse, so that it may be something very fugitive the bad effects of which will quickly disappear or something which becomes as serious, as grave as it can be. I don't know if you have noticed that there are people who never miss the opportunity of an accident! Every time there is the possibility of an accident, they have it. And never is their accident ordinary. Every time the accident can be serious, it is serious. Well, usually in life one says: "Oh! he is unlucky, he is unfortunate, indeed he has no luck." But all that is ignorance. It depends absolutely on the working of his consciousness. I could give you examples — only I would have to speak about certain people and I don't want to. But I could give you striking examples! And this — this is the sort of thing one sees all the time, all the time here! There are people who could have been killed and who come out of it unscathed; there are others for whom it was not serious, and it becomes serious.

But that does not depend on thought, on the working of the ordinary thought. They may apparently have thoughts as good as the others — it is not that. It is the second of the choice — people knowing how to react just in the right way at the right time. I could give you hundreds of examples. It is quite interesting.

This depends absolutely on character. Some have such an awakened consciousness, so alert, that they are not asleep, they are awake within. Just at the second it is required they call the help. Or they invoke the divine Force. But just at the second it is needed. So the danger is averted, nothing happens. They could have been killed: they come out of it absolutely unhurt. Others, on the contrary, as soon as they have the least little scratch, something gets dislocated in their being: a sort of fright or pessimism or defeatism in their consciousness which automatically comes up — it was nothing, they had just twisted their leg and the next minute they break it. There is no reason for it. They could very well have not broken their leg.

There are others who climb up to a first floor on a ladder which gives way under them. They could have collapsed — they come out of that without the least hurt. How did they manage it? Apparently this seems wonderful, and still this is how things happen to them. They find themselves lying on the ground in an altogether fine state; nothing has happened to them. I could give you the names, I am telling you exact facts.

So, on what does this depend? It depends on whether one is sufficiently awake for the second of the choice to... And note that this is not at all mental, it is not that: it is an attitude of the being, it is the consciousness reacting in the right way. It goes quite far, very far, it is formidable, the power of this attitude. But as it is just a fraction of a second, it implies an altogether awakened consciousness which never sleeps, never enters the inconscient. For one does not know when these things are going to happen, isn't that so? Hence, one does not have the time to wake up. One must be awake.

I knew someone who, indeed, should have died and did not die because of this. For his consciousness reacted very fast. He had taken poison by mistake: instead of taking one dose of a certain medicine, he had taken twelve and it was a poison; he should have died, the heart should have stopped (it was many years ago) and he is still quite alive! He reacted in the right way.

If these things were narrated they would be called miracles. They are not miracles: it is an awakened consciousness.

How were we saved the other day when working down there with the crane?[1]

[1] A team of young Ashram disciples was trying to lift a tree-trunk

I suppose you ought to know!

We know partly.

Very partially, vaguely, a sort of impression "like that" — an impression, almost an attitude, but not knowledge. How that works, one would not be able to say!

It was by grace.

But if you can explain to me how that works, it would be interesting for everybody. It would be very interesting to know who exactly had that wakeful consciousness, had faith and a sort of... something that answered automatically, and perhaps not consciously.

There are degrees, many degrees. Human intelligence is such that unless there is a contrast it does not understand. You know, I have received hundreds of letters from people thanking me because they had been saved; but it is very, very rarely that someone writes to thank me because nothing has happened, you understand! Let us take an accident, it is already the beginning of a disorder. Naturally when it is a public or collective accident, the atmosphere of each person has its part in the thing, and that depends on the proportion of defeatists and those who, on the contrary, are on the right side. I don't know if I have written this — it is written somewhere — but it is a very interesting thing. I am going to tell

---

into a truck with the help of a crane, when the crane broke apart, flying into pieces on all sides, but without hurting anyone. Then the tree-trunk, half lifted in, began rolling slowly, causing the truck to lean on one side threatening to crush several boys, when, without any apparent reason or any physical object to hold it back, the trunk suddenly stopped in its course.

you.... People are not aware of the workings of grace except when there has been some danger, that is, when there has been the beginning of an accident or the accident has taken place and they have escaped it. Then they become aware. But never are they aware that if, for instance, a journey or anything whatever, passes without any accident, it is an infinitely higher grace. That is, the harmony is established in such a way that nothing can happen. But that seems to them quite natural. When people are ill and get well quickly, they are full of gratitude; but never do they think of being grateful when they are well; and yet that is a much greater miracle! In collective accidents, what is interesting is exactly the proportion, the sort of balance or disequilibrium, the combination made by the different atmospheres of people.

There was an aviator, one of the great "aces", as they are called, of the First [World] War, and a marvellous aviator. He had gained numerous victories, nothing had ever happened to him. But something occurred in his life and suddenly he felt that something was going to happen to him, an accident, that it was now all over. What they call their "good luck" had gone. This man left the military to enter civil aviation and he piloted one of these lines — no, not civil aviation: he came out of the war but remained with the military planes. And then he wanted to make a trip to South Africa: from France to South Africa. Evidently, something must have been upset in his consciousness (I did not know him personally, so I don't know what happened). He started from a certain city in France to go to Madagascar, I believe (I am not sure, I think it was Madagascar). And from there he wanted to come back to France. My brother was at that time governor of the Congo, and he wanted to get back quickly to his post. He asked to be allowed as a passenger on the plane (it was one of those planes for professional tours, to show what these planes could do). Many people wanted to dissuade my brother from going by it; they told him, "No, these trips are always dangerous, you must not go on them." But finally he went all the same. They had a breakdown and stopped in the middle of the Sahara, a situation not very pleasant. Yet everything was arranged as by a miracle, the plane started again and put down my brother in the Congo, exactly where he wanted to go, then it went farther south. And soon after, half-way the plane crashed — and the other man was killed.... It was obvious that this had to happen. But my brother had an absolute faith in his destiny, a certitude that nothing would happen. And it was translated in this way: the mixture of the two atmospheres made the dislocation unavoidable, for there was a breakdown in the Sahara and the plane was obliged to land, but finally everything was in order and there was no real accident. But once he was no longer there, the other man had all the force of his "ill-luck" (if you like), and the accident was complete and he was killed.

A similar incident happened to a boat. There were two persons (they were well-known people but I cannot remember their names now), who had gone to Indo-China by plane. There was an accident, they were the only ones to have been saved, all the others were killed, indeed it was quite a dramatic affair. But these two (husband and wife) must have been what may be called bringers of bad-luck — it is a sort of atmosphere they carry. Well, these two wanted to go back to France (for, in fact, the accident occurred on their way back to France), they wanted to return to France, they took a boat. And quite unexpectedly, unusually, right in the midst of the Red Sea the boat ran into a reef (a thing that doesn't happen even once in a million voyages) and sank; and the others were drowned, and these two were saved. And I could do nothing, you know, I wanted to say: "Take care, never travel with these people!"...

There are people of this sort, wherever they are they come out of the thing very well, but the catastrophes are for the others.

If one sees things from the ordinary viewpoint, one does not notice this. But the associations of atmosphere — one must take care of that. That is why when one travels in groups, one must know with whom one travels. One should have an inner knowledge, should have a vision. And then, if one sees somebody who has a kind of small black cloud around him, one must take care not to travel with him; for, surely an accident will occur — though perhaps not to him. Hence, it is quite useful to know things a little more deeply than in the altogether superficial way.

23 December 1953

8

DOCTORS AND MEDICINES

Doctors Are Soldiers, Doctors Are Priests

Truth is supreme harmony and supreme delight.

All disorder, all suffering is falsehood.

Thus it can be said that illnesses are the falsehoods of the body, and consequently doctors are soldiers of the great and noble army fighting in the world for the conquest of Truth.

*

If the body is considered as the tabernacle of the Lord, then medical science, for example, becomes the initiatory ritual for temple service and doctors of all categories are priests officiating in the different rituals of the worship. Thus medicine is truly a priesthood and should be treated as such.

The same thing may be said of physical culture and all sciences dealing with the body and its working. And if the material universe is regarded as the external robe and manifestation of the Supreme, then it can be said, generally, that all physical sciences are rituals of worship.

*

A broad mind, a generous heart, an unflinching will, a quiet, steady determination, an inexhaustible energy and a total trust in one's mission — this makes a perfect doctor.

*

To medical knowledge and experience, add full faith in the Divine's Grace and your healing capacity will have no limits.

*

After all, an illness is only a wrong attitude taken by some part of the body.

The chief role of the doctor is, by various means, to induce the body to recover its trust in the Supreme Grace.

*

My dear child, I quite agree with you that there is a power other and much more powerful than that of the doctors and the medicines and I am glad to see that you put your trust in it. Surely it will lead you through all difficulties and in spite of catastrophic warnings. Keep your faith intact and all will be all right.

*

It is true that the faith cures more than the treatment. You might take Dr. S's treatment and call for the Divine's help.

*

The only thing I can suggest about diseases is to call down peace. Keep the mind away from the body by whatever means — whether by reading Sri Aurobindo's books or meditation. It is in this state that the Grace acts. And it is the Grace alone that cures. The medicines only give a faith to the body. That is all.

*

In every case, it is the Force that cures.

Medicines have little effect; it is faith in medicine that cures.

Let the doctor whom you trust treat you and take only the medicines that you feel you can trust.

The body only has trust in material methods, that is why you have to give it medicine — but medicine only has an effect if the Force acts through it.

*

The whole value of a medicine is in the Spirit it contains.

*

My advice is that medicines should not be used unless it is absolutely impossible to avoid them; and this "absolutely impossible" should be very strict.

Medicines Are Not All-powerful

If a certain medicine, through a concurrence of favourable circumstances, has cured a number of people, immediately it is proclaimed that this medicine is all-powerful against this disease. But it is not true. And the proof is that if the same medicine is administered in the same way to a hundred people, there won't be two similar results, and sometimes the effects will be diametrically opposite. Therefore, it is not the property of the medicine itself which cures; to believe in this medicine is a superstition.

14 March 1956

Medicines Help the Body to Have Confidence

Mother, how are medicines to be used for a body which is not altogether unconscious? For even when we draw on the divine grace, we see that we need a little medicine, and if a little medicine is given it has a good effect. Does this mean that only the body needs medicine or is there something wrong with the mind and the vital?

In most cases the use of medicines — within reasonable limits, that is, when one doesn't poison oneself by taking medicines — is simply to help the body to have confidence. It is the body which heals itself. When it wants to be cured, it is cured. And this is something very widely recognised now; even the most traditional doctors tell you, "Yes, our medicines help, but it is not the medicines which cure, it is the body which decides to be cured." Very well, so when the body is told, "Take this", it says to itself, "Now I am going to get better", and because it says "I am going to get better", well, it is cured!

In almost every case, there are things which help — a little — provided it is done within reasonable limits. If it is no longer within reasonable limits, you are sure to break down completely. You cure one thing but catch another which is usually worse. But still, a little help, in a way, a little something that gives confidence to your body: "Now it will be all right, now that I have taken this, it is going to be all right" — this helps it a great deal and it decides to get better and it is cured.

There too, there is a whole range of possibilities, from the yogi who is in so perfect a state of inner control that he could take poison without being poisoned to the one who at the least little scratch rushes to the doctor and needs all sorts of special drugs to get his body to make the movement needed for its cure. There is the whole possible range, from total, supreme mastery to an equally total bondage to all external aids and all that you absorb from outside — a bondage and a perfect liberation. There is the whole range. So everything is possible. It is like a great key-board, very complex and very complete, on which one can play, and the body is the instrument.

19 June 1957

Medical Knowledge

About medical knowledge in the world: if you have studied enough or lived long enough, that is, a fairly good number of years, you will find that with the same authority, the same certitude, the same conviction, at one time certain things are not only considered bad, but on the basis of an absolute knowledge, an unquestionable observation, they are reputed to have a certain effect, and at another time these very unquestionable observations lead to diametrically opposite results. Very often I give an example which I happened to observe, especially as regards the value of certain foods and their effects on the body, like certain fruits or vegetables: at a particular time in medical history — not so long ago, about fifty or sixty years ago — when you had a certain illness, the doctor gave you a list of things recommending to you with absolute seriousness not to touch any of these lest you become even more ill — I could give you the list, but it is not interesting. Well, about these very same things, fifty or sixty years later, not the same doctor perhaps but another one will tell you with the same seriousness, the same unquestionable certitude and authority that these are the very things you must eat if you want to be cured! So if you have observed things pretty well and have a slightly critical mind, you can tell yourself, "Oh! it must depend on people or perhaps on the period." And I shall tell you, as the doctor-friend I knew in France forty or fifty years ago used to tell all his patients, "Take a remedy while it is in fashion, for then it will cure you."

21 November 1956

A Doctor's Advice

I knew a doctor who was a neuropath and treated illnesses of the stomach. He used to say that all illnesses of the stomach came from a more or less bad nervous state. He was a doctor for the rich and it was the rich and unoccupied people who went to him. So they used to come and tell him: "I have a pain in the stomach, I cannot digest", and this and that. They had terrible pains, they had headache, they had, well, all the phenomena! He used to listen to them very seriously. I knew a lady who went to him and to whom he said: "Ah! your case is very serious. But on which floor do you live? on the groundfloor? All right. This is what you have to do to cure your illness of the stomach. Take a bunch of fully ripe grapes (do not take your breakfast, for breakfast upsets your stomach), take a bunch of grapes; hold it in your hand, like this, very carefully. Then prepare to go out — not by your door, never go out by your door! You must go out by the window. Get a stool. And go out by the window. Go out in the street, and there you must walk while eating one grape every two steps — not more, yes, not more! You will have stomach-ache! One single grape every two steps. You must take two steps, then eat one single grape and you should continue till there are no more grapes. Do not turn back, go straight on till there are no more grapes. You must take a big bunch. And when you have finished, you may return quietly. But do not take a conveyance! Come back on foot, otherwise the whole trouble will return. Come back quietly and I give you the guarantee that if you do that every day, at the end of three days you will be cured." And in fact this lady was cured!

24 June 1953

9

SPIRITUAL CURE OF OTHERS

Forces That Act for Healing

The power of formation has a great advantage, if one knows
how to use it. You can make good formations and if you
make them properly, they will act in the same way as the
others. You can do a lot of good to people just by sitting
quietly in your room, perhaps even more good than by under-
going a lot of trouble externally. If you know how to think cor-
rectly, with force and intelligence and kindness, if you love
someone and wish him well very sincerely, deeply, with all
your heart, that does him much good, much more certainly
than you think. I have said this often; for example, to those
who are here, who learn that someone in their family is very
ill and feel that childish impulse of wanting to rush immediately to the spot to attend to the sick person. I tell you,
unless it is an exceptional case and there is nobody to attend
on the sick person (and at times even in such a case), if you
know how to keep the right attitude and concentrate with
affection and good will upon the sick person, if you know how
to pray for him and make helpful formations, you will do
him much more good than if you go to nurse him, feed him,
help him wash himself, indeed all that everybody can do.
Anybody can nurse a person. But not everybody can make
good formations and send out forces that act for healing.

1 July 1953

Re-establish Equilibrium by an Inner Power

In reality illness is only a disequilibrium; if then you are able to establish another equilibrium, this disequilibrium disappears. An illness is simply, always, in every case, even when the doctors say that there are microbes — in every case, a disequilibrium in the being: a disequilibrium among the various functions, a disequilibrium among the forces.

This is not to say that there are no microbes: there are, there are many more microbes than are known now. But it is not because of that you are ill, for they are always there. It happens that they are always there and for days they do nothing to you and then all of a sudden, one day, one of them gets hold of you and makes you ill — why? Simply because the resistance was not as it used to be habitually, because there was some disequilibrium in some part, the functioning was not normal. But if, by an inner power, you can re-establish the equilibrium, then that's the end, there is no more difficulty, the disequilibrium disappears.

There is no other way of curing people. It is simply when one sees the disequilibrium and is capable of re-establishing the equilibrium that one is cured. Only there are two very different categories you come across. Some hold on to their disequilibrium — they hold on to it, cling to it, don't want to let it go. Then you may try as hard as you will, even if you re-establish the equilibrium the next minute they get into disequilibrium once again, because they love that. They say: "Oh no! I don't want to be ill", but within them there is something which holds firmly to some disequilibrium, which does not want to let it go. There are other people, on the contrary, who sincerely love equilibrium, and directly you give them the power to get back their equilibrium, the equilibrium is re-established and in a few minutes they are cured. Their knowledge was not sufficient or their power was not sufficient to re-establish order — disequilibrium is a disorder. But if you intervene, if you have the knowledge and re-establish the equilibrium, quite naturally the illness will disappear; and those who allow you to do it get cured. Only those who do not let you do it are not cured and this is visible, they do not allow you to act, they cling to the illness. I tell them: "Ah! you are not cured? Go to the doctor then." And the funniest part of the thing is that most often they believe in the doctors, although the working remains the same! Every doctor who is something of a philosopher will tell you: "It is like that; we doctors give only the occasion, but it is the body that cures itself. When the body wants to be cured, it is cured." Well, there are bodies that do not allow equilibrium to be re-established unless they are made to absorb some medicine or something very definite which gives them the feeling that they are being truly looked after. But if you give them a very precise, very exact treatment that is sometimes very difficult to follow, they begin to be convinced that there is nothing better to do than to regain the equilibrium and they get back the equilibrium!

24 June 1953

Curing an Illness Spiritually

Once, I complained to you about some pain and you asked me which part of the body was affected. When I told you which, I did not know about its correspondence with the vital, the mind, etc., yet the pain disappeared.

I don't see any contradiction!... There are two ways of curing an illness spiritually. One consists in putting a force of consciousness and truth on the physical spot which is affected. In this case the effect produced depends naturally on the receptivity of the person. Supposing the person is receptive; the force of consciousness is put upon the affected part and its pressure restores order. . . .

In other cases, if the body lacks receptivity altogether or if its receptivity is insufficient, one sees the inner correspondence with the psychological state which has brought about the illness and acts on that. But if the cause of the illness is refractory, not much can be done. Let us say the origin is vital. The vital absolutely refuses to change, it clings terrifically to the condition in which it is; then that is hopeless. You put the force, and usually it provokes an increase in the illness, produced by the resistance of the vital which did not want to accept anything. I speak of the vital but it can be the mind or something else.

When the action is directly upon the body, that is, on the affected part, it is possible that one is relieved; then, some hours later or even after a few days, the illness returns. This means that the cause has not been changed, that the cause is in the vital and is still there; it is only the effect which has been cured. But if one can act simultaneously upon both the cause and the effect, and the cause is sufficiently receptive to consent to change, then one is completely cured, once for all.

31 March 1951

Cure by the Mother's Grace: Each Case Is Different

Mother, I am asking you a small personal question. An incurable illness, an organic disease has been cured by your grace, but a purely functional illness is not. How can that be? In the same body. Is it a lack of receptivity or...?

It is something so personal, so individual, that it is impossible to reply. As I said, for each one the case is absolutely different, and one can't give an explanation for these things without going into the details of the functioning. For each one, the case is different.

And for every thing, every event, there are so many explanations as there are planes of consciousness. In a way... well, in an over-simplified way, one may say that there is a physical explanation, a vital explanation, a mental explanation, a spiritual explanation, there is... there is an entire gradation of countless explanations that you could give for the same phenomenon. None is altogether true, all have an element of truth. And finally, if you want to enter the field of explanations, if you take one thing and follow it up, you always have to explain it by another, and you may go round the world indefinitely and explain one thing by another without ever reaching the end of your explanation.

Indeed, when one sees this in its totality and its essence, the wisest thing one can say is: "It is like that because it is like that."

19 June 1957

The Mother's Intervention to Cure

When people are taken ill or when they are caught in an accident, well, whether I see it myself or come to know of it from outside through someone's telling me about it — in every case it is not the same. There are cases when I am informed and I see that it is for intervening and I have the full power to change the consequence, that is, to cure the sick person. There are cases where I see I am not to intervene. For instance, it is time for the person to quit his body: he will leave the body. But knowing this, I must do for the person and for his environment

what has to be done for the event to have the maximum beneficial effect or the minimum adverse effect — it depends on the
circumstances.

29 July 1953

Sri Aurobindo Performed Miracles in the Mind

*"The supernatural is that the nature of which we have not
attained or do not yet know, or the means of which we have
not yet conquered. The common taste for miracles is the sign
that man's ascent is not yet finished.*

*"It is rationality and prudence to distrust the super-
natural; but to believe in it is also a sort of wisdom.*

*"Great saints have performed miracles; greater saints
have railed at them; the greatest have both railed at them
and performed them.*

*"Open thy eyes and see what the world really is and
what God; have done with vain and pleasant imaginations."*

Sri Aurobindo, Thoughts and Aphorisms

*Why didn't you or Sri Aurobindo make a greater use of
miracles as a means of overcoming resistance in the external human consciousness ? Why this kind of self-effacement
where outer things are concerned, this non-intervention
or discretion ?*

As for Sri Aurobindo, I only know what he told me several
times. People give the name of "miracle" only to interventions
in the material or the vital world. And these interventions are
always mixed with ignorant and arbitrary movements.

But the number of miracles that Sri Aurobindo performed

in the mind is incalculable; but naturally you could only see it if you had a very straight, very sincere, very pure vision — a few people did see it. But he refused — this I know — he refused to perform any vital or material miracles, because of this mixture. . . .

I did not quite understand what you meant by saying that Sri Aurobindo performed miracles in the mind.

I mean that he used to introduce the supramental force into the mental consciousness. Into the mental consciousness, the mental consciousness that governs all material movements, he would introduce a supramental formation or power or force which immediately changed the organisation. This produces immediate effects which seem illogical because they do not follow the normal course of movements according to mental logic.

He himself used to say that when he was in possession of the supramental power, when he could use it at will and focus it on a specific point with a definite purpose, it was irrevocable, inevitable: the effect was absolute. That can be called a miracle.

For example, take someone who was sick or in pain; when Sri Aurobindo was in possession of this supramental power — there was a time when he said that it was completely under his control, that is, he could do what he wanted with it, he could apply it where he liked — then he would apply this Will, for example, to some disorder, either physical or vital or, of course, mental — he would apply this force of greater harmony, of greater order, this supramental force, and focus it there, and it would act immediately. And it was an order: it created an order, a harmony greater than the natural harmony. That is, if it was a case of healing, for example, the healing would be more perfect and more complete than any obtained by ordinary physical and mental methods.

There were a great many of them. But people are so blind, so embedded in their ordinary consciousness that they always give "explanations", they can always give an explanation. Only those who have faith and aspiration and something very pure in themselves, that is, who truly want to know, they were able to perceive it.

When the Power was there, he even used to say that it was effortless; all he had to do was to apply this supramental power of order and harmony and instantly the desired result was achieved.

6 March 1963

Cure by Sri Aurobindo

One follows the place in one's head where the little point [of troublesome thoughts] is dancing. I have seen — I have seen Sri Aurobindo doing this in somebody's head, somebody who used to complain of being troubled by thoughts. It was as if his hand reached out and took hold of the little black dancing point and then did this (*gesture with the finger-tips*), as when one picks up an insect, and he threw it far away. And that was all. All still, quiet, luminous.... It was clearly visible like this, you know, he took it out without saying anything — and it was over.

And things are very closely interdependent: I also saw the case when someone came to him with an acute pain somewhere: "Oh! it hurts here, oh! it hurts, oh!..." He said nothing, he remained calm, he looked at the person, and I saw, I saw something like a subtle physical hand which came and took hold of the little point dancing about in disorder and confusion, and he took it like this (*same gesture*) and there, everything had gone.

"Oh! oh! look my pain has gone."

8 January 1958

10

HYPNOTISM

Hypnotism: A Modernised Form of Occultism

Now they are finding out that they can replace anæsthetics by hypnotism with infinitely better results. Well, hypnotism is a form — a form modernised in its expression — of occultism; a very limited, very small form of a very tiny power compared with occult power, but still it is a form of occultism which has been put in modern terms to make the thing modern. And I don't know if you have heard about these things, but they are very interesting from a certain point of view: for instance, this process of hypnotism has been tried on someone who had to have a skin-graft on a wound. I don't remember all the details now, but the arm had to remain attached to the leg for a fortnight.... If the person were immobilised by plaster and bandages and all sorts of things, at the end of the fortnight he wouldn't be able to move — everything would become stiff and he would need weeks of treatment to recover the free use of his arm. In this case, nothing was tied up, nothing was physically immobilised — no plaster, no bandages, nothing — the person was just hypnotised and told to keep his arm in that position. He kept it for a fortnight, without any effort, any difficulty, without any intervention from his will: it was the will of the hypnotiser which intervened. It was perfectly successful, the arm remained in the required position, and when the fortnight was over and the hypnotism removed, and the person was told, "Now you may move", he began to move! Well, that's a step forward.

Sweet Mother, they say hypnotism has a bad after-effect on the hypnotised person?

No, no! If somebody practises hypnotism to impose his will on another, it can obviously do much harm to the other person, but we are speaking of a hypnotism which is practised in a humanitarian way, it might be said, and for precise reasons. All the bad effects can be avoided if the one who does it has no bad intentions.

If you use chemical formulas in an ignorant way, you can cause an explosion (*laughter*), and that is very dangerous! Well, if you use occult formulas ignorantly — or egoistically, which is even worse than ignorantly — you can also have harmful results. But that doesn't mean that occultism is bad or hypnotism is bad or chemistry is bad. You are not going to ban chemistry because there are people who cause explosions! (*Laughter*)

10 September 1958

II

PAIN AND SUFFERING

Do Not Cherish Suffering

One cannot help others to overcome their griefs and sufferings unless one overcomes them in oneself and becomes master of one's sentiments and reactions.

*

My word to you is: Do not cherish suffering and suffering will leave you altogether. Suffering is far from being indispensable to progress. The greatest progress is made through a steady and cheerful equanimity.

*

If you make one mistake in life, then you may have to suffer all your life. It does not mean that everybody suffers like that. There are people who go on making mistakes and yet they do not suffer. But those who are born for a spiritual life have to be very careful.

*

Do not take the sorrows of life for what they seem to be — they are in truth a way to greater achievements.

To Know How to Suffer

If at any time a deep sorrow, a searing doubt or an intense pain overwhelms you and drives you to despair, there is an infallible way to regain calm and peace.

In the depths of our being there shines a light whose brilliance is equalled only by its purity; a light, a living and conscious portion of a universal godhead who animates and nourishes and illumines Matter, a powerful and unfailing guide for those who are willing to heed his law, a helper full of solace and loving forbearance towards all who aspire to see and hear and obey him. No sincere and lasting aspiration towards him can be in vain; no strong and respectful trust can be disappointed, no expectation ever deceived.

My heart has suffered and lamented, almost breaking beneath a sorrow too heavy, almost sinking beneath a pain too strong.... But I have called to thee, O divine comforter, I have prayed ardently to thee, and the splendour of thy dazzling light has appeared to me and revived me.

As the rays of thy glory penetrated and illumined all my being, I clearly perceived the path to follow, the use that can be made of suffering; I understood that the sorrow that held me in its grip was but a pale reflection of the sorrow of the earth, of this abysm of suffering and anguish.

Only those who have suffered can understand the suffering of others; understand it, commune with it and relieve it. And I understood, O divine comforter, sublime Holocaust, that in order to sustain us in all our troubles, to soothe all our pangs, thou must have known and felt all the sufferings of earth and man, all without exception.

How is it that among those who claim to be thy worshippers, some regard thee as a cruel torturer, as an inexorable judge witnessing the torments that are tolerated by thee or even created by thy own will?

No, I now perceive that these sufferings come from the very imperfection of Matter which, in its disorder and crudeness, is unfit to manifest thee; and thou art the very first to suffer from it, to bewail it, thou art the first to toil and strive in thy ardent desire to change disorder into order, suffering into happiness, discord into harmony.

Suffering is not something inevitable or even desirable, but when it comes to us, how helpful it can be!

Each time we feel that our heart is breaking, a deeper door opens within us, revealing new horizons, ever richer in hidden treasures, whose golden influx brings once more a new and intenser life to the organism on the brink of destruction.

And when, by these successive descents, we reach the veil that reveals thee as it is lifted, O Lord, who can describe the intensity of Life that penetrates the whole being, the radiance of the Light that floods it, the sublimity of the Love that transforms it for ever!

1910

The Secret towards Which Pain Leads Us

"Pain and grief are Nature's reminder to the soul that the pleasure it enjoys is only a feeble hint of the real delight of existence. In each pain and torture of our being is the secret of a flame of rapture compared with which our greatest pleasures are only as dim flickerings. It is this secret which forms the attraction for the soul of the great ordeals, sufferings and fierce experiences of life which the nervous mind in us shuns and abhors."

Sri Aurobindo, Thoughts and Glimpses

Quite naturally we ask ourselves what this secret is, towards which pain leads us. For a superficial and imperfect understanding, one could believe that it is pain which the soul is seeking. Nothing of the kind. The very nature of the soul is divine Delight, constant, unvarying, unconditioned, ecstatic; but it is true that if one can face suffering with courage, endurance, an unshakable faith in the divine Grace, if one can, instead of shunning suffering when it comes, enter into it with this will, this aspiration to go through it and find the luminous truth, the unvarying delight which is at the core of all things, the door of pain is often more direct, more immediate than that of satisfaction or contentment.

I am not speaking of pleasure because pleasure turns its back constanly and almost completely on this profound divine Delight.

Pleasure is a deceptive and perverse disguise which turns us away from our goal and we certainly should not seek it if we are eager to find the truth. Pleasure vaporises us; it deceives us, leads us astray. Pain brings us back to a deeper truth by obliging us to concentrate in order to be able to bear it, be able to face this thing that crushes us. It is in pain that one most easily finds the true strength again, when one is strong. It is in pain that one most easily finds the true faith again, the faith in something which is above and beyond all pain.

When one enjoys oneself and forgets, when one takes things as they come, tries to avoid being serious and looking life in the face, in a word when one seeks to forget, to forget that there is a problem to solve, that there is something to find, that we have a reason for existence and living, that we are not here just to pass our time and go away without having learnt or done anything, then one really wastes one's time, one misses the opportunity that has been given to us, this — I cannot say unique, but marvellous opportunity for an existence which is the field of progress, which is the moment in eternity when you can discover the secret of life; for this physical, material existence is a wonderful opportunity, a possibility given to you to find the purpose of life, to make you advance one step towards this deeper truth, to make you discover this secret which puts you into contact with the eternal rapture of the divine. life.

(Silence)

I have already told you many a time that to seek suffering and pain is a morbid attitude which must be avoided, but to run away from them through forgetfulness, through a superficial, frivolous movement, through diversion, is cowardice. When pain comes, it comes to teach us something. The quicker we learn it, the more the need for pain diminishes, and when we know the secret, it will no longer be possible to suffer, for that secret reveals to us the reason, the cause, the origin of suffering, and the way to pass beyond it.

The secret is to emerge from the ego, get out of its prison, unite ourselves with the Divine, merge into Him, not to allow anything to separate us from Him. Then, once one has discovered this secret and realises it in one's being, pain loses its justification and suffering disappears. It is an all-powerful remedy, not only in the deeper parts of the being, in the soul, in the spiritual consciousness, but also in life and in the body.

There is no illness, no disorder which can resist the discovery of this secret and the putting of it into practice, not only in the higher parts of the being but in the cells of the body.

If one knows how to teach the cells the splendour that lies within them, if one knows how to make them understand the reality which makes them exist, gives them being, then they too enter the total harmony, and the physical disorder which causes the illness vanishes as do all other disorders of the being.

But for that one must be neither cowardly nor fearful. When the physical disorder comes, one must not be afraid; one must not run away from it, must face it with courage, calmness, confidence, with the certitude that illness is a *falsehood* and that if one turns entirely, in full confidence, with a complete quietude to the divine Grace, It will settle in these cells as It is established in the depths of the being, and the cells themselves will share in the eternal Truth and Delight.

13 February 1957

Teach the Body to Bear Pain

Pain is the touch of our Mother teaching us how to bear and grow in rapture. She has three stages of her schooling, endurance first, next equality of soul, last ecstasy.

Sri Aurobindo, Thoughts and Aphorisms

As far as moral things are concerned, this is absolutely obvious, it is indisputable — all moral suffering moulds your character and leads you straight to ecstasy, when you know how to take it. But when it comes to the body...

It is true that doctors have said that if one can teach the body to bear pain, it becomes more and more resilient and less easily disrupted — this is a concrete result. In the case of people who know how to avoid getting completely upset as soon as they have a pain somewhere, who are able to bear it quietly, to keep their balance, it seems that the body's capacity to bear the disorder without going to pieces increases. This is a great achievement. I had asked myself this question from the purely practical, external standpoint and it seems to be like this. Inwardly, I had been told this many times — told and shown by small experiences — that the body can bear much more than we think, if no fear or anxiety is added to the pain. If we eliminate the mental factor, the body, left to itself, has neither fear nor apprehension nor anxiety about what is going to happen — no anguish — and it can bear a great deal.

The second step is when the body has decided to bear it — you see, it takes the decision to bear it: immediately, the acuteness, what is acute in the pain disappears. I am speaking absolutely materially.

And if you are calm — here, another factor comes in, the need for inner calm — if you have the inner calm, then the pain changes into an almost pleasant sensation — not "pleasant" in the ordinary sense, but an almost comfortable feeling comes. Again, I am speaking purely physically, materially.

And the last stage, when the cells have faith in the divine Presence and in the sovereign divine Will, when they have this trust that all is for the good, then ecstasy comes — the cells open, like this, become luminous and ecstatic.

That makes four stages — only three are mentioned here.

The last one is probably not within everyone's reach, but the first three are quite evident — I *know* it is like that. The only thing that used to worry me was that it was not a purely psychological experience and that there was some wear in the body by the fact of enduring suffering. But I have asked doctors and I was told that if the body is taught to bear pain when it is very young, its capacity to endure increases so much that it can really resist disease; that is, the disease does not follow its normal course, it is arrested. That is precious.

10 August 1963

Turn the Consciousness Upward

You may have been told that certain bodily complaints will give you a great deal of pain. Things like that are often said. You then make a formation of fear and keep expecting the pain. And the pain comes even when it need not.

But in case it is there after all, I can tell you one thing. If the consciousness is turned upward, the pain vanishes. If it is turned downward, the pain is felt and even increases. When one experiments with the upward and the downward turnings, one sees that the bodily complaint as such has nothing to do with the pain. Although the body may suffer very much or not at all, its condition may be exactly the same. It is the turn of the consciousness that makes all the difference.

I say "turned upward", because to turn towards the Divine is the best method, but what can be said in general is that if the consciousness is turned away from the pain to one's work or anything that interests one, the pain ceases.

And not only the pain but whatever damage there may be in an organ is set right much more easily when the consciousness is taken away from the trouble and one is open to the Divine. There is the *Sat* aspect of the Divine — the pure supreme Existence above or beyond or behind the cosmos. If you can keep in contact with it, all physical complaints can be removed.

25 Novemeber 1962

Accustom the Body to Understand

When there is a clearly localised illness in the body, what is the best way of opening the physical consciousness to receive the healing Force?

For this — as for everything else in this domain which may be called the "outposts" of occultism or the threshold of occultism — each one must find his own movement; for what is most effective for each one is the method for which he has been more or less prepared and which is most familiar to him. So it is very difficult to make a general rule.

But there is a preparation which may be of a general kind. That is, to accustom the body methodically to understand that it is only the outer expression of a truer and deeper reality and that it is this truer and deeper reality which governs its destiny — though it is not usually aware of it.

One can prepare the body through a series of observations, studies, understandings[1], by showing it examples, making it understand things as one makes a child understand them, either by observing its own movements — but generally, in this, one is comparatively blind! — or by observing those of others. And in a more general way, this preparation will be based on recognised studies, on clear facts. Like this, for instance: that a certain number of persons, placed in exactly similar circumstances, experience, each one of them, very different effects. One may go even further: in a given set of definite circumstances, there is a certain number of particular, definite individuals, in apparently quite identical conditions, and for some the effects are catastrophic, while others escape without any harm.

During the war there was a very large number of such examples for study. In epidemics it is the same thing; in cataclysms of Nature, like tidal waves or earthquakes or cyclones, it is the same thing.

The body understands these things if they are shown and

---

[1] For the body, to understand is to have the capacity of execution, obtained through the contagion of example. For, "to understand" for the body means to be able to do. (Mother's note)

explained to it as one explains things to a child: "You see, there was something *else* that acted there, not only the plain material fact by itself." And, unless some bad will is there, it understands.

This is a preparation.

Gradually, if you make use of this understanding, you must, with a methodical work of infusing consciousness into the cells of the body, infuse at the same time the truth of the divine Presence. This work takes time, but, if done methodically and constantly, it produces an effect.

So you have prepared the ground.

Suppose that as a result of some illness or other, there is some sort of pain at a precise spot. At that moment all will depend, as I said at the beginning, on the approach most familiar to you. But we can give an example. You are in pain, in great pain; it is hurting very much, you are suffering a lot.

First point: do not stress the pain by telling yourself, "Oh, how painful! Oh, this pain is unbearable! Oh, it is becoming worse and worse, I shall never be able to bear it", etc., all this sort of thing. The more you go on thinking like this and feeling like this and the more your attention is concentrated on it, the pain increases amazingly.

So, the first point: to control yourself sufficiently not to do that.

Second point: as I said, it depends on your habits. If you know how to concentrate, to be quiet, and if you can bring into yourself a certain peace, of any kind — it may be a mental peace, it may be a vital peace, it may be a psychic peace; they have different values and qualities, this is an individual question — you try to realise within yourself a state of peace or attempt to enter into a conscious contact with a force of peace.... Suppose you succeed more or less completely.

Then, if you can draw the peace into yourself and bring it down into the solar plexus — for we are not talking of inner states but of your physical body — and from there direct it very calmly, very slowly I might say, but very persistently, towards the place where the pain is more or less sharp, and fix it there, this is very good.

This is not always enough.

But if by widening this movement you can add a sort of mental formation with a little life in it — not just cold, but with a little life in it — that the only reality is the divine Reality, and all the cells of this body are a more or less deformed expression of this divine Reality — there is only one Reality, the Divine, and our body is a more or less deformed expression of this sole Reality — if by my aspiration, my concentration, I can bring into the cells of the body the consciousness of this *sole* Reality, all disorder must necessarily cease.

If you can add to that a movement of complete and trusting surrender to the Grace, then I am sure that within five minutes your suffering will disappear. If you know how to do it.

You may try and yet not succeed. But you must know how to try again and again and again, until you do succeed. But if you do those three things at the same time, well, there is no pain which can resist.

4 July 1956

Develop the Faculty of Reason

One may have sufferings and not feel them, be as if they did not exist. That is, a misfortune, a "cross" touches only the outer consciousness, the physical, the mental, the vital, but the psychic — in truth, the psychic is above all suffering. Let us take a very simple example: an illness. A physical disorder brings suffering, at times much suffering, but there are people who are in such a state of consciousness that their physical sufferings do not exist, they are not real for them. It is the same thing with separation; if you love someone and are separated from that person, you suffer — this is one of the most common of sufferings, it is the ties which are broken — well, in a certain state of consciousness the real link between two beings cannot be broken, for it does not belong to the domain where things break. Therefore one is above what may happen.

But before one reaches a higher state of consciousness, there is a stage where one can develop in oneself the faculty of reason — a clear, precise, logical reason, sufficiently objective in its vision of things. And when one has developed this reason well, all impulses, feelings, desires, all disturbances can be put in the presence of this reason and that makes you reasonable. Most people, when something troubles them, become very unreasonable. When, for example, they are ill, they pass their time saying, "Oh, how ill I am, how frightful it is; is it going to last like that all the time?" And naturally it gets worse and worse. Or when some misfortune befalls them, they cry out: "It is only to me that these things happen and I was thinking that everything was fine before", and they burst into a fit of tears, a fit of nerves. Well, not to speak of superman, in man himself there is a higher capacity called reason, which is able to look at things calmly, coolly, reasonably. And this reason tells you, "Don't worry, that will improve nothing, you must not grumble, you must accept the thing since it has come." Then you immediately become calm. It is a very good mental training, it develops judgment, vision, objectivity and at the same time it has a very healthy action upon your character. It helps you to avoid the ridiculousness of giving way to your nerves and lets you behave like a reasonable person.

20 January 1951

Eliminating Pain

Physical sufferings? One thing is certain, you know; I think this was in the system, in the nature, that it [suffering] was invented as an indicator; because, for example, if the body was disorganised in some way or other and this caused no suffering at all, one would never look for a way to stop the disorganisation. One thinks of curing an illness only because one suffers. If it caused you no unpleasantness, you would never think of being cured of it. So, in the economy of Nature I think that the first purpose of physical suffering was to give you a warning.

Unfortunately, there is the vital which pokes its nose into the affair and takes a very perverse pleasure in increasing, twisting, sharpening the suffering. Now this deforms the whole system because instead of being an indicator, sometimes it becomes an occasion for enjoying the illness, for making oneself interesting, and also having the opportunity to pity oneself — all kinds of things which all come from the vital and are all detestable, one more than another. But ordinarily I think that it was this: "Take care." You see, it's like a danger-signal: "Take care, there's something out of order."

Only, when one is not very much coddled, when one has a little endurance and decides within himself not to pay too much attention, quite remarkably the pain diminishes. And there are a number of illnesses or states of physical imbalance which can be cured simply by removing the effect, that is, by stopping the suffering. Usually it comes back because the cause is still there. If the cause of the illness is found and one acts directly on its cause, then one can be cured radically. But if one is not able to do that, one can make use of this influence, of this control over pain in order — by cutting off the pain or eliminating it or mastering it in oneself — to work on the illness. So this is an effect, so to say, from outside inwards; while the other is an effect from within outwards, which is much more lasting and much more complete. But the other also is effective.

For example, you see, some people suffer from unbearable toothache. It depends above all... some people are more or less what I call "coddled", that is, unable to resist any pain, to bear it; they immediately say, "I can't! It is unbearable. I can't bear any more!" Ah, this indeed changes nothing in the circumstances; it does not stop the suffering, because it is not by telling it that you don't want it that you make it go away. But if one can do two things: either bring into oneself — for all nervous suffering, for example — bring into oneself a kind of immobility, as total as possible, at the place of pain, this has the effect of an anaesthetic. If one succeeds in bringing an inner immobility, an immobility of the inner vibration, at the spot where one is suffering, it has exactly the same effect as an anaesthetic. It cuts off the contact between the place of pain and the brain, and once you have cut the contact, if you can keep this state long enough, the pain will disappear. You must form the habit of doing this. But you have the occasion, all the time, the opportunity to do it: you get a cut, get a knock, you see, one always gets a little hurt somewhere — especially when doing athletics, gymnastics and all that — well, these are opportunities given to us. Instead of sitting there observing the pain, trying to analyse it, concentrating upon it, which makes it increase indefinitely... (There are people who think of something else but it does not last; they think of something else and then suddenly are drawn back to the place that hurts.) But if one can do this... You see, since the pain is there, it proves that you are in contact with the nerve that's transmitting the pain, otherwise you wouldn't feel it. Well, once you know that you are in contact, you try to accumulate at that point as much immobility as you can, to stop the vibration of the pain; you will perceive then that it has the effect of a limb which goes to sleep when you are in an awkward position and that all of a sudden... you know, don't you?... and then, when it stops, it begins to vibrate again terribly. Well, you deliberately try this kind of concentration of immobility in the painful nerve; at the painful point you bring as total an immobility as you can. Well, you will see that it works, as I told you, like an anaesthetic: it puts the thing to sleep. And then, if you can add to that a kind of inner peace and a trust that the pain will go away, well, I tell you that it will go.

Of all things, that which is considered the most difficult from the yogic point of view is toothache, because it is very close to the brain. Well, I know that this can be done truly to the extent of not feeling the pain at all; and this does not cure the bad tooth, but there are cases in which one can succeed in killing the painful nerve. Usually in a tooth it is the nerve which has been attacked by the caries, the disease, and which begins to protest with all its strength. So, if you succeed in establishing this immobility, you prevent it from vibrating, you prevent it from protesting. And what is remarkable is that if you do it fairly constantly, with sufficient perseverance, the sick nerve will die and you will not suffer at all any more. Because it was that which was suffering and when it is dead it does not suffer any longer. Try. I hope you never have a toothache. (*Laughter*)

17 November 1954

FEAR OF DEATH

Remedies: Reason, Find the Psychic Being

Mother, sometimes we are terribly afraid. What should we do in such a case?

Ah! that depends on the nature of the fear. Is it a fear without a cause or is it based on a cause? Because the remedy differs.

It is based on a cause.

Ah! For example, when someone is ill, one is afraid of catching the illness. . . .

No, someone is dead.

And one is afraid to die.

There are two remedies. There are many, but two at least are there. In any case, the use of a deeper consciousness is essential. One remedy consists in saying that it is something that happens to everyone (let us take it on that level), yes, it is a thing that happens to everybody, and therefore, sooner or later, it will come and there is no reason why one should be afraid, it is quite a normal thing. You may add one more idea to this, that according to experience (not yours but just the collective human experience), circumstances being the same, absolutely identical, in one case people die, in another they do not — why? And if you push the thing a little further still, you say to yourself that after all it must depend on something which is altogether outside your consciousness — and in the end one dies when one has to die. That is all. When one has to die one dies, and when one has not to die, one does not die. Even when you are in mortal danger, if it is not your hour to die, you will not die, and even if you are out of all danger, just a scratch on your foot will be enough to make you die, for there are people who have died of a pin-scratch on the foot — because the time had come. Therefore, fear has no sense. What you can do is to rise to a state of consciousness where you can say, "It is like that, we accept the fact because it seems to be recognised as an inevitable fact. But I do not need to worry, for it will come only when it must come. So I don't need to feel afraid: when it is not to come, it will not come to me, but when it must come to me, it will come. And as it will come to me inevitably, it is better I do not fear the thing; on the contrary, one must accept what is perfectly natural." This is a well-known remedy, that is to say, very much in use.

There is another, a little more difficult, but better, I believe. It lies in telling oneself: "This body is not I", and in trying to find in oneself the part which is truly one's self, until one has found one's psychic being. And when one has found one's psychic being — immediately, you understand — one has the sense of immortality. And one knows that what goes out or what comes in is just a matter of convenience: "I am not going to weep over a pair of shoes I put aside when it is full of holes! When my pair of shoes is worn out I cast it aside, and I do not weep." Well, the psychic being has taken this body because it needed to use it for its work, but when the time comes to leave the body, that is to say, when one must leave it because it is no longer of any use for some reason or other, one leaves the body and has no fear. It is quite a natural gesture — and it is done without the least regret, that's all.

And the moment you are in your psychic being, you have

that feeling, spontaneously, effortlessly. You soar above the physical life and have the sense of immortality. As for me, I consider this the best remedy. The other is an intellectual, commonsense, rational remedy. This is a deep experience and you can always get it back as soon as you recover the contact with your psychic being. This is a truly interesting phenomenon, for it is automatic. The moment you are in contact with your psychic being, you have the feeling of immortality, of having always been and being always, eternally. And then what comes and goes — these are life's accidents, they have no importance. Yes, this is the best remedy. The other is like the prisoner finding good reasons for accepting his prison. This one is like a man for whom there's no longer any prison. . . .

Now, there is a small remedy which is very very easy. For it is based on a simple personal question of one's common sense.... You must observe yourself a little and say that when you are afraid it is as though the fear was attracting the thing you are afraid of. If you are afraid of illness, it is as though you were attracting the illness. If you are afraid of an accident, it is as though you were attracting the accident. And if you look into yourself and around yourself a little, you will find it out, it is a persistent fact. So if you have just a little common sense, you say: "It is stupid to be afraid of anything, for it is precisely as though I were making a sign to that thing to come to me. If I had an enemy who wanted to kill me, I would not go and tell him: 'You know, it's me you want to kill!' " It is something like that. So, since fear is bad, we won't have it. And if you say you are unable to prevent it by your reason, well, that shows you have no control over yourselves and must make a little effort to control yourselves. That is all.

Oh! There are many ways of curing oneself of fear. But in

reality everyone finds his own way, the one good for him. There are people to whom you have simply to say: "Your fear is a weakness", and they would immediately find the means to look at it with contempt, for they have a horror of weakness. There are others, you tell them: "Fear is a suggestion from hostile forces, you must push it away, as you drive off hostile forces", and this is very effective. For each one it is different. But first of all you must know that fear is a very bad thing, very bad, it is a dissolvent; it is like an acid. If you put a drop of it on something, it eats into the substance. The first step is not to admit the possibility of fear. Yes, that's the first step. I knew people who used to boast about their fear. These are incurable. That is, quite naturally they would say, "Ah, just imagine, I was so frightened!" And then what! It is nothing to be proud of. With such people you can do nothing.

However, when once you recognise that fear is neither good nor favourable nor noble nor worthy of a consciousness a little enlightened, you begin to fight against it. And I say, one man's way is not another's; one must find one's own way; it depends on each one. Fear is also a terribly contagious collective thing — contagious, it is much more catching than the most contagious of illnesses. You breathe an atmosphere of fear and instantly you feel frightened, without even knowing why or how, nothing, simply because there was an atmosphere of fear. A panic at an accident is nothing but an atmosphere of fear spreading round over everybody. And it is quite curable. There have been numerous cases of a panic being stopped outright simply because some people refused the suggestion and could counteract it with an opposite suggestion. For mystics the best cure as soon as one begins to feel afraid of something is to think of the Divine and then snuggle in his arms or at his feet and leave him entirely responsible for everything that happens, within, outside, everywhere — and immediately the fear disappears. That is the cure for the mystic. It is the easiest of all. But everybody does not enjoy the grace of being a mystic.

14 October 1953

Remedies: Reason, Inner Seeking, Trust in God

The first method [to overcome the fear of death] appeals to the reason. One can say that in the present state of the world, death is inevitable; a body that has taken birth will necessarily die one day or another, and in almost every case death comes when it must: one can neither hasten nor delay its hour. Someone who craves for it may have to wait very long to obtain it and someone who dreads it may suddenly be struck down in spite of all the precautions he has taken. The hour of death seems therefore to be inexorably fixed, except for a very few individuals who possess powers that the human race in general does not command. Reason teaches us that it is absurd to fear something that one cannot avoid. The only thing to do is to accept the idea of death and quietly do the best one can from day to day, from hour to hour, without worrying about what is going to happen. This process is very effective when it is used by intellectuals who are accustomed to act according to the laws of reason; but it would be less successful for emotional people who live in their feelings and let themselves be ruled by them. No doubt, these people should have recourse to the second method, the method of inner seeking. Beyond all the emotions, in the silent and tranquil depths of our being, there is a light shining constantly, the light of the psychic consciousness. Go in search of this light, concentrate on it; it is within you. With a persevering will, you are sure to find it and as soon as you enter into it, you awake to the sense of immortality. You have always lived, you will always live; you become wholly independent of your body; your conscious existence does not depend on it; and this body is only one of the transient forms through which you have manifested. Death is no longer an extinction, it is only a transition. All fear instantly vanishes and you walk through life with the calm certitude of a free man.

The third method is for those who have faith in a God, their God, and who have given themselves to him. They belong to him integrally; all the events of their lives are an expression of the divine will and they accept them not merely with calm submission but with gratitude, for they are convinced that whatever happens to them is always for their own good. They have a mystic trust in their God and in their personal relationship with him. They have made an absolute surrender of their will to his and feel his unvarying love and protection, wholly independent of the accidents of life and death. They have the constant experience of lying at the feet of their Beloved in an absolute self-surrender or of being cradled in his arms and enjoying a perfect security. There is no longer any room in their consciousness for fear, anxiety or torment; all that has been replaced by a calm and delightful bliss.

Bulletin, February 1954

PART III

FOUNDATIONS OF HEALTH

GOOD HABITS

We Must Protect Happiness and Good Health

As yet happiness and good health are not normal conditions in this world.

We must protect them very carefully against the intrusion of their opposites.

*

It is only by correcting your ways of living that you can hope to secure good health.

*

Do not forget that to succeed in our yoga we must have a strong and healthy body.

For that, the body must do exercise, have an active and regular life, eat well, do physical work and sleep well.

It is in good health that the way towards transformation is found.

*

It is good to do exercises and to lead a simple and hygienic life, but for the body to be truly perfect, it must open to the divine forces, it must be subject only to the divine influence, it must aspire constantly to realise the Divine.

Why Doctors, Dispensaries, Physical Education?

I have often been asked this question, "Why, after having posited as an ideal principle that when we deal with our body we ought to do it with the knowledge that it is only a result and an instrument of the supreme Reality of the universe and of the truth of our being, — why, after having taught this and shown that this is the truth to be realised, do we have, in the organisation of our Ashram, doctors, dispensaries, a physical education of the body based on modern theories accepted everywhere?" And why, when some of you go for a picnic do I forbid you to drink water from just anywhere and tell you to take filtered water with you? Why do I have the fruit you eat disinfected, etc.?

All this seems contradictory, but this evening I intend to explain something to you which, I hope, will put an end to this feeling of a contradiction in you. In fact, I have told you many a time that when two ideas or principles apparently seem to contradict one another, you must rise a little higher in your thought and find the point where the contradictions meet in a comprehensive synthesis.

Here, it is very easy if we know one thing, that the method we use to deal with our body, maintain it, keep it fit, improve it and keep it in good health, depends *exclusively* on the state of consciousness we are in; for our body is an instrument of our consciousness and this consciousness can act directly on it and obtain what it wants from it.

So, if you are in an ordinary physical consciousness, if you see things with the eyes of the ordinary physical consciousness, if you think of them with the ordinary physical consciousness, it will be ordinary physical means you will have to use to act on your body. These ordinary physical means make up the whole science which has accumulated through thousands of years of human existence. This science is very complex, its processes innumerable, complicated, uncertain, often contradictory, always progressive and almost absolutely relative! Still, very precise results have been achieved; ever since physical culture has become a serious preoccupation, a certain number of experiments, studies, observations have accumulated, which enable us to regulate diet, activities, exercise, the whole outer organisation of life, and provide an adequate basis so that those who make the effort to study and conform strictly to these things have a chance to maintain their body in good health, correct the defects it may have and improve its general condition, and even achieve results which are sometimes quite remarkable.

I may add, moreover, that this intellectual human science, such as it is at present, in its very sincere effort to find the truth, is, surprisingly enough, drawing closer and closer to the essential truth of the Spirit. It is not impossible to foresee the movement where the two will unite in a very deep and very close understanding of the essential truth.

So, for all those who live on the physical plane, in the physical consciousness, it is physical means and processes which have to be used in dealing with the body. And as the vast majority of human beings, even in the Ashram, live in a consciousness which, if not exclusively physical, is at least predominantly physical, it is quite natural for them to follow and obey all the principles laid down by physical science for the care of the body.

29 May 1957

Physical Education

Of all the domains of human consciousness, the physical is the one most completely governed by method, order, discipline, process. The lack of plasticity and receptivity in matter has to be replaced by a detailed organisation that is both precise and comprehensive. In this organisation, one must not forget the interdependence and interpenetration of all the domains of the being. However, even a mental or vital impulse, to express itself physically, must submit to an exact process. That is why all education of the body, if it is to be effective, must be rigorous and detailed, far-sighted and methodical. This will be translated into habits; the body is a being of habits. But these habits should be controlled and disciplined, while remaining flexible enough to adapt themselves to circumstances and to the needs of the growth and development of the being.

All education of the body should begin at birth and continue throughout life. It is never too soon to begin nor too late to continue.

Physical education has three principal aspects: (1) control and discipline of the functioning of the body, (2) an integral, methodical and harmonious development of all the parts and movements of the body and (3) correction of any defects and deformities.

It may be said that from the very first days, even the first hours of his life, the child should undergo the first part of this programme as far as food, sleep, evacuation, etc. are concerned. If the child, from the very beginning of his existence, learns good habits, it will save him a good deal of trouble and inconvenience for the rest of his life; and besides, those who have the responsibility of caring for him during his first years will find their task very much easier.

Naturally, this education, if it is to be rational, enlightened and effective, must be based upon a minimum knowledge of the human body, of its structure and its functioning. As the child develops, he must gradually be taught to observe the functioning of his internal organs so that he may control them more and more, and see that this functioning remains normal and harmonious. As for positions, postures and movements, bad habits are formed very early and very rapidly, and these may have disastrous consequences for his whole life. Those who take the question of physical education seriously and wish to give their children the best conditions for normal development will easily find the necessary indications and instructions. The subject is being more and more thoroughly studied, and many books have appeared and are still appearing which give all the information and guidance needed.

It is not possible for me here to go into the details of the application, for each problem is different from every other and the solution should suit the individual case. The question of food has been studied at length and in detail; the diet that helps children in their growth is generally known and it may be very useful to follow it. But it is very important to remember that the instinct of the body, so long as it remains intact, is more reliable than any theory. Accordingly, those who want their child to develop normally should not force him to eat food which he finds distasteful, for most often the body possesses a sure instinct as to what is harmful to it, unless the child is particularly capricious.

The body in its normal state, that is to say, when there is no intervention of mental notions or vital impulses, also knows very well what is good and necessary for it; but for this to be effective in practice, one must educate the child with care and teach him to distinguish his desires from his needs. He should be helped to develop a taste for food that is simple and healthy, substantial and appetising, but free from any useless complications. In his daily food, all that merely stuffs and causes heaviness should be avoided; and above all, he must be taught to eat according to his hunger, neither more nor less, and not to make his meals an occasion to satisfy his greed or gluttony. From one's very childhood, one should know that one eats in order to give strength and health to the body and not to enjoy the pleasures of the palate. Children should be given food that suits their temperament, prepared in a way that ensures hygiene and cleanliness, that is pleasant to the taste and yet very simple. This food should be chosen and apportioned according to the age of the child and his regular activities. It should contain all the chemical and dynamic elements that are necessary for his development and the balanced growth of every part of his body.

Since the child will be given only the food that helps to keep him healthy and provide him with the energy he needs, one must be very careful not to use food as a means of coercion and punishment. The practice of telling a child, "You have not been a good boy, you won't get any dessert," etc., is most harmful. In this way you create in his little consciousness the impression that food is given to him chiefly to satisfy his greed and not because it is indispensable for the proper functioning of his body.

Another thing should be taught to a child from his early years: to enjoy cleanliness and observe hygienic habits. But, in obtaining this cleanliness and respect for the rules of hygiene from the child, one must take great care not to instil into him the fear of illness. Fear is the worst instrument of education and the surest way of attracting what is feared. Yet, while there should be no fear of illness, there should be no inclination for it either. There is a prevalent belief that brilliant minds are found in weak bodies. This is a delusion and has no basis. There was perhaps a time when a romantic and morbid taste for physical unbalance prevailed; but, fortunately, that tendency has disappeared. Nowadays a well-built, robust, muscular, strong and well-balanced body is appreciated at its true value. In any case, children should be taught to respect health and admire the healthy man whose vigorous body knows how to repel attacks of illness. Often a child feigns illness to avoid some troublesome obligation, a work that does not interest him, or simply to soften his parents' hearts and get them to satisfy some caprice. The child must be taught as early as possible that this does not work and that he does not become more interesting by being ill, but rather the contrary. The weak have a tendency to believe that their weakness makes them particularly interesting and to use this weakness and if necessary even illness as a means of attracting the attention and sympathy of the people around them. On no account should this pernicious tendency be encouraged. Children should therefore be taught that to be ill is a sign of weakness and inferiority, not of some virtue or sacrifice.

That is why, as soon as the child is able to make use of his limbs, some time should be devoted every day to the methodical and regular development of all the parts of his body. Every day some twenty or thirty minutes, preferably on waking, if possible, will be enough to ensure the proper functioning and balanced growth of his muscles while preventing any stiffening of the joints and of the spine, which occurs much sooner than one thinks. In the general programme of the child's education, sports and outdoor games should be given a prominent place; that, more than all the medicines in the world, will assure the child good health. An hour's moving about in the sun does more to cure weakness or even anæmia than a whole arsenal of tonics. My advice is that medicines should not be used unless it is absolutely impossible to avoid them; and this "absolutely impossible" should be very strict. In this programme of physical culture, although there are well-known general lines to be followed for the best development of the human body, still, if the method is to be fully effective in each case, it should be considered individually, if possible with the help of a competent person, or if not, by consulting the numerous manuals that have already been and are still being published on the subject.

But in any case a child, whatever his activities, should have a sufficient number of hours of sleep. The number will vary according to his age. In the cradle, the baby should sleep longer than he remains awake. The number of hours of sleep will diminish as the child grows. But until maturity it should not be less than eight hours, in a quiet, well-ventilated place. The child should never be made to stay up late for no reason. The hours before midnight are the best for resting the nerves. Even during the waking hours, relaxation is indispensable for all who want to maintain their nervous balance. To know how to relax the muscles and the nerves is an art which should be taught to children when they are very young. There are many parents who, on the contrary, push their child to constant activity. When the child remains quiet, they imagine that he is ill. There are even parents who have the bad habit of making their child do household work at the expense of his rest and relaxation. Nothing is worse for a developing nervous system, which cannot stand the strain of too continuous an effort or of an activity that is imposed upon it and not freely chosen. At the risk of going against many current ideas and ruffling many prejudices, I hold that it is not fair to demand service from a child, as if it were his duty to serve his parents. The contrary would be more true, and certainly it is natural that parents should serve their child or at least take great care of him. It is only if a child chooses freely to work for his family and does this work as play that the thing is admissible. And even then, one must be careful that it in no way diminishes the hours of rest that are absolutely indispensable for his body to function properly.

I have said that from a young age children should be taught to respect good health, physical strength and balance. The great importance of beauty must also be emphasised. A young child should aspire for beauty, not for the sake of pleasing others or winning their admiration, but for the love of beauty itself; for beauty is the ideal which all physical life must realise. Every human being has the possibility of establishing harmony among the different parts of his body and in the various movements of the body in action. Every human body that undergoes a rational method of culture from the very beginning of its existence can realise its own harmony and thus become fit to manifest beauty. When we speak of the other aspects of an integral education, we shall see what inner conditions are to be fulfilled so that this beauty can one day be manifested.

So far I have referred only to the education to be given to children for a good many bodily defects can be rectified and many malformations be avoided by an enlightened physical education given at the proper time. But if for any reason this physical education has not been given during childhood or even in youth, it can begin at any age and be pursued throughout life. But the later one begins, the more one must be prepared to meet bad habits that have to be corrected, rigidities to be made supple, malformations to be rectified. And this preparatory work will require much patience and perseverance before one can start on a constructive programme for the harmonisation of the form and its movements. But if you keep alive within you the ideal of beauty that is to be realised, sooner or later you are sure to reach the goal you have set yourself.

Bulletin, April 1951

The Discipline of Beauty

The tapasya or discipline of beauty will lead us, through austerity in physical life, to freedom in action. Its basic programme will be to build a body that is beautiful in form, harmonious in posture, supple and agile in its movements, powerful in its activities and robust in its health and organic functioning.

To achieve these results, it will be good, as a general rule, to make use of habit as a help in organising one's material life, for the body functions more easily within the framework of a regular routine. But one must know how to avoid becoming a slave to one's habits, however good they may be; the greatest flexibility must be maintained so that one may change them each time it becomes necessary to do so.

One must build up nerves of steel in powerful and elastic muscles in order to be able to endure anything whenever it is indispensable. But at the same time great care must be taken not to demand more from the body than the effort which is strictly necessary, the expenditure of energy that fosters growth and progress, while categorically excluding everything that causes exhaustion and leads in the end to physical decline and disintegration.

A physical culture which aims at building a body capable of serving as a fit instrument for a higher consciousness demands very austere habits: a great regularity in sleep, food, exercise and every activity. By a scrupulous study of one's own bodily needs — for they vary with each individual — a general programme will be established; and once this has been done well, it must be followed rigorously, without any fantasy or slackness. There must be no little exceptions to the rule that are indulged in "just for once" but which are repeated very often — for as soon as one yields to temptation, even "just for once", one lessens the resistance of the will-power and opens the door to every failure. One must therefore forego all weakness: no more nightly escapades from which one comes back exhausted, no more feasting and carousing which upset the normal functioning of the stomach, no more distractions, amusements and pleasures that only waste energy and leave one without the strength to do the daily practice. One must submit to the austerity of a sensible and regular life, concentrating all one's physical attention on building a body that comes as close to perfection as possible. To reach this ideal goal, one must strictly shun all excess and every vice, great or small; one must deny oneself the use of such slow poisons as tobacco, alcohol, etc., which men have a habit of developing into indispensable needs that gradually destroy the will and the memory. The all-absorbing interest which nearly all human beings, even the most intellectual, have in food, its preparation and its consumption, should be replaced by an almost chemical knowledge of the needs of the body and a very scientific austerity in satisfying them. Another austerity must be added to that of food, the austerity of sleep. It does not consist in going without sleep but in knowing how to sleep. Sleep must not be a fall into unconsciousness which makes the body heavy instead of refreshing it. Eating with moderation and abstaining from all excess greatly reduces the need to spend many hours in sleep; however, the quality of sleep is much more important than its quantity. In order to have a truly effective rest and relaxation during sleep, it is good as a rule to drink something before going to bed, a cup of milk or soup or fruit-juice, for instance. Light food brings a quiet sleep. One should, however, abstain from all copious meals, for then the sleep becomes agitated and is disturbed by nightmares, or else is dense, heavy and dulling. But the most important thing of all is to make the mind clear, to quieten the emotions and calm the effervescence of desires and the preoccupations which accompany them. If before retiring to bed one has talked a lot or had a lively discussion, if one has read an exciting or intensely interesting book, one should rest a little without sleeping in order to quieten the mental activity, so that the brain does not engage in disorderly movements while the other parts of the body alone are asleep. Those who practise meditation will do well to concentrate for a few minutes on a lofty and restful idea, in an aspiration towards a higher and vaster consciousness. Their sleep will benefit greatly from this and they will largely be spared the risk of falling into unconsciousness while they sleep.

After the austerity of a night spent wholly in resting in a calm and peaceful sleep comes the austerity of a day which is sensibly organised; its activities will be divided between the progressive and skilfully graded exercises required for the culture of the body, and work of some kind or other. For both can and ought to form part of the physical tapasya. With regard to exercises, each one will choose the ones best suited to his body and, if possible, take guidance from an expert on the subject, who knows how to combine and grade the exercises to obtain a maximum effect. Neither the choice nor the execution of these exercises should be governed by fancy. One must not do this or that because it seems easier or more amusing; there should be no change of training until the instructor considers it necessary. The self-perfection or even simply the self-improvement of each individual body is a problem to be solved, and its solution demands much patience, perseverance and regularity. In spite of what many people think, the athlete's life is not a life of amusement or distraction; on the contrary, it is a life of methodical efforts and austere habits, which leave no room for useless fancies that go against the result one wants to achieve.

In work too there is an austerity. It consists in not having any preferences and in doing everything one does with interest. For one who wants to grow in self-perfection, there are no great or small tasks, none that are important or unimportant; all are equally useful for one who aspires for progress and self-mastery. It is said that one only does well what one is interested in doing. This is true, but it is truer still that one can learn to find interest in everything one does, even in what appear to be the most insignificant chores. The secret of this attainment lies in the urge towards self-perfection. Whatever occupation or task falls to your lot, you must do it with a will to progress; whatever one does, one must not only do it as best one can but strive to do it better and better in a constant effort for perfection. In this way everything without exception becomes interesting, from the most material chore to the most artistic and intellectual work. The scope for progress is infinite and can be applied to the smallest thing.

This leads us quite naturally to liberation in action. For, in one's action, one must be free from all social conventions, all moral prejudices. However, this does not mean that one should lead a life of licence and dissoluteness. On the contrary, one imposes on oneself a rule that is far stricter than all social rules, for it tolerates no hypocrisy and demands a perfect sincerity. One's entire physical activity should be organised to help the body to grow in balance and strength and beauty. For this purpose, one must abstain from all pleasure-seeking, including sexual pleasure. For every sexual act is a step towards death. That is why from the most ancient times, in the most sacred and secret schools, this act was prohibited to every aspirant towards immortality. The sexual act is always followed by a longer or shorter period of unconsciousness that opens the door to all kinds of influences and causes a fall in consciousness. But if one wants to prepare oneself for the supramental life, one must never allow one's consciousness to slip into laxity and inconscience under the pretext of pleasure or even of rest and relaxation. One should find relaxation in force and light, not in darkness and weakness. Continence is therefore the rule for all those who aspire for progress. But especially for those who want to prepare themselves for the supramental manifestation, this continence must be replaced by a total abstinence, achieved not by coercion and suppression but by a kind of inner alchemy, as a result of which the energies that are normally used in the act of procreation are transmuted into energies for progress and integral transformation. It is obvious that for the result to be total and truly beneficial, all sexual impulses and desires must be eliminated from the mental and vital consciousness as well as from the physical will. All radical and durable transformation proceeds from within outwards, so that the external transformation is the normal, almost inevitable result of this process.

A decisive choice has to be made between lending the body to Nature's ends in obedience to her demand to perpetuate the race as it is, and preparing this same body to become a step towards the creation of the new race. For it is not possible to do both at the same time; at every moment one has to decide whether one wants to remain part of the humanity of yesterday or to belong to the superhumanity of tomorrow.

One must renounce being adapted to life as it is and succeeding in it if one wants to prepare for life as it will be and to become an active and efficient part of it.

One must refuse pleasure if one wants to open to the delight of existence, in a total beauty and harmony.

Bulletin, February 1953

2

REST, SLEEP AND DREAMS

Proper Rest: Important for the Sadhana

Proper rest is a very important thing for the sadhana.

*

You must *rest* — but a rest of *concentrated force*, not of diluted non-resistance to the adverse forces. A rest that is *a power*, not the rest of weakness.

*

Before going to sleep, when you lie down to sleep, begin by relaxing yourself physically (I call this becoming a rag on the bed).

Then with all the sincerity at your disposal offer yourself to the Divine in a complete relaxation, and... that's all.

Keep trying until you succeed and you will see.

*

I would like to know why I had such a disturbed night.

Obviously you did not quiet your thoughts before going to sleep. At the time of lying down one should always begin by quieting one's thoughts.

*

Sleep is indispensable in the present state of the body. It is by a progressive control over the subconscient that the sleep can become more and more conscious.

*

I know by experience that it is not by lessening the food that the sleep becomes conscious; the body becomes restless but in no way it increases the consciousness. It is in a good, sound and quiet sleep that one can get in contact with a deeper part of oneself.

Rest in Action

"The body has a wonderful capacity of adaptation and endurance. It is fit to do so many more things than one can usually imagine. If instead of the ignorant and despotic masters that govern it, it is ruled by the central truth of the being, one will be surprised at what it is capable of doing. Calm and quiet, strong and poised, it will at every minute put forth the effort that is demanded of it, for it will have learnt to find rest in action, to recuperate through contact with the universal forces the energies it spends consciously and usefully."

The Mother, *"The Science of Living"*

How can one have "rest in action"?

That comes from a kind of certitude of inner choice. When one aspires for something, if at the same time one knows that the aspiration will be heard and answered in the best way possible, that establishes a quietude in the being, a quietude in its vibrations; whilst if there is a doubt, an uncertainty, if one does not know what will lead one to the goal or if ever one will reach it or whether there is a way of doing so, and so on, then one gets disturbed and that usually creates a sort of little whirlwind around the being, which prevents it from receiving the real thing. Instead, if one has a quiet faith, if whilst aspiring one knows that there is no aspiration (naturally, sincere aspiration) which remains unanswered, then one is quiet. One aspires with as much fervour as possible, but does not stand in nervous agitation asking oneself why one does not get immediately what one has asked for. One knows how to wait. I have said somewhere: "To know how to wait is to put time on one's side." That is quite true. For if one gets excited, one loses all one's time — one loses one's time, loses one's energy, loses one's movements. To be very quiet, calm, peaceful, with the faith that what is true will take place, and that if one lets it happen, it will happen so much the quicker. Then, in that peace everything goes much better.

16 December 1953

Try Not to Think of Anything

This [identifying yourself] is also one of the methods used today to cure nervous diseases. When someone cannot sleep, cannot be restful because he is too excited and nervous and his nerves are ill and weakened by excessive agitation, he is told to sit in front of an aquarium, for instance — an aquarium, that's very lovely, isn't it? — before an aquarium with pretty little fish in it, goldfish; just to sit there, settle down in an easy-chair and try not to think of anything (particularly not of his troubles) and look at the fish. So he looks at the fish, moving around, coming and going, swimming, gliding, turning, meeting, crossing, chasing one another indefinitely, and also the water flowing slowly and the passing fish. After a while he lives the life of fishes: he comes and goes, swims, glides, plays. And at the end of the hour his nerves are in a perfect state and he is completely restful!

But the condition is that one must not think of one's troubles, simply watch the fish.

12 August 1953

Relax, Widen, Call the Peace

How can one increase the receptivity of the body?

It depends on the part. The method is almost the same for all parts of the being. To begin with, the first condition: to remain as quiet as possible. You may notice that in the different parts of your being, when something comes and you do not receive it, this produces a shrinking — there is something which hardens in the vital, the mind or the body. There is a stiffening and this hurts, one feels a mental, vital or physical pain. So, the first thing is to put one's will and relax this shrinking, as one does a twitching nerve or a cramped muscle; you must learn how to relax, be able to relieve this tension in whatever part of the being it may be.

The method of relaxing the contraction may be different in the mind, the vital or the body, but logically it is the same thing. Once you have relaxed the tension, you see first if the disagreeable effect ceases, which would prove that it was a small momentary resistance, but if the pain continues and if it is indeed necessary to increase the receptivity in order to be able to receive what is helpful, what should be received, you must, after having relaxed this contraction, begin trying to widen yourself — you feel your are widening yourself. There are many methods. Some find it very useful to imagine they are floating on water with a plank under their back. Then they widen themselves, widen, until they become the vast liquid mass. Others make an effort to identify themselves with the

sky and the stars, so they widen, widen themselves, identi-
fying themselves more and more with the sky. Others again
don't need these pictures; they can become conscious of their
consciousness, enlarge their consciousness more and more
until it becomes unlimited. One can enlarge it till it becomes
vast as the earth and even the universe. When one does that
one becomes really receptive. As I have said, it is a question of
training. In any case, from an immediate point of view, when
something comes and one feels that it is too strong, that it
gives a headache, that one can't bear it, the method is just the
same, you must act upon the contraction. One can act through
thought, by calling the peace, tranquillity (the feeling of peace
takes away much of the difficulty) like this: "Peace, peace,
peace... tranquillity... calm." Many discomforts, even physical, like all these contractions of the solar plexus, which are
so unpleasant and give you at times nausea, the sensation of
being suffocated, of not being able to breathe again, can
disappear thus. It is the nervous centre which is affected,
it gets affected very easily. As soon as there is something
which affects the solar plexus, you must say, "Calm... calm...
calm", become more and more calm until the tension is
destroyed.

In thought also. For instance, you are reading something
and come across a thought you don't understand — it is beyond you, you understand nothing and so in your head it lies
like a brick, and if you try to understand, it becomes more and
more like a brick, a stiffening, and if you persist it gives you
a headache. There is but one thing to do: not to struggle
with the words, remain just like this (*gesture: stretched out,
immobile*), create a relaxation, simply widen, widen. And don't
try to understand, above all, don't try to understand — let it
enter like that, quite gently, and relax, relax, and in this relaxing your headache goes away. You no longer think of any-

thing, you wait for a few days and after some days you see from inside: "Oh! how clear it is! I understand what I had not understood." It is as easy as that.

31 March 1951

Relax, Give Yourself, Repeat Your Mantra

Why does one get up tired in the morning, and what should one do to have better sleep?

If you get up tired in the morning, it is because of *tamas*, nothing else, a formidable mass of tamas; I discovered it when I began to do the yoga of the body. It is inevitable so long as the body is not transformed.

You must lie flat on your back and relax all the muscles and nerves — it is an easy thing to learn — to be like what I call a piece of cloth on the bed; nothing else remains. If you can do that with the mind also, you get rid of all the stupid dreams that make you more tired when you get up than when you went to bed. It is the cellular activity of the brain that continues without control, and that tires much. Therefore a total relaxation, a kind of complete calm, without tension in which everything is stopped. But this is only the beginning.

Afterwards, a self-giving as total as possible, of all, from top to bottom, from the outside to the inmost, and an eradication also as total as possible of all resistance of the ego, and you begin repeating your mantra — your mantra, if you have one or any other word which has power over you, a word leaping from the heart, spontaneously, like a prayer and that sums up your aspiration. After having repeated a few times, if you are accustomed to it, you get into trance. And from that trance you pass into sleep. The trance lasts as long as it should and quite naturally, spontaneously you pass into sleep. But when you come back from this sleep, you remember everything, the sleep was but a continuation of the trance.

Fundamentally the sole purpose of sleep is to enable the body to assimilate the effect of the trance so that the effect may be accepted everywhere, to enable the body to do its natural function of the night and eliminate the toxins. And when it wakes up, there is no trace of heaviness which comes from sleep, the effect of the trance continues.

Even for those who have never been in trance, it is good to repeat a mantra, a word, a prayer before going into sleep. But there must be a life in the words, I do not mean an intellectual signification, nothing of that kind, but a vibration. And on the body its effect is extraordinary: it begins to vibrate, vibrate, vibrate... and quietly you let yourself go as though you wanted to get into sleep. The body vibrates more and more and still more and away you go. That is the cure for tamas.

It is tamas which causes bad sleep. There are two kinds of bad sleep: the sleep that makes you heavy, dull, as though you lose all the effect of the effort you put in during the preceding day; and the sleep that exhausts you as if you were passing your time in fight. I have noticed that if you cut your sleep into slices (it is simply a habit to form), the nights become better. That is to say, you must be able to come back to your normal consciousness and aspiration at fixed intervals — come back to the call of the consciousness... but for that you must not make use of an alarm bell. When you are in trance, it is not good to be shaken out of it.

When you are about to go into sleep, you can make a formation and say "I shall wake up at such an hour" (you do that very well when you are a child). For the first stretch of sleep you must count at least three hours; for the last one hour is sufficient. But the first one must be three hours at the minimum. On the whole, you have to remain in bed at least seven hours; in six hours you do not have time enough to do much (naturally I am looking from the point of view of sadhana) to make the nights useful.

To make use of the nights is an excellent thing; it has a double effect: a negative effect, it prevents you from falling backward, losing whatever you have gained — that, indeed, is painful — and a positive effect, you make some progress, you continue your progress. You make use of the night; then there is no trace of fatigue any more.

Two things you must eliminate: falling into the torpor of the inconscience, with all these things of the subconscient and of the inconscient that rise up, invade you, enter into you; and a vital and mental superactivity where you pass your time in fighting, literally, terrible battles. People come out of that state bruised, as if they had received blows — and they did receive them; then it is not "as if"! And I see only one way, change the nature of sleep.

Relax, Make Your Brain Silent and Immobile

There is no end to the discoveries that one can make in dreams. But one thing is very important: never go to sleep when you are very tired, for if you do that you fall into a kind of inconscience and dreams do with you whatever they like without your being able to exercise the least control. Just as you should always take rest before you eat, I would advise you all to rest before you go to sleep. But you must know how to rest.

There are many ways of doing it. Here is one: first of all, repose your body, comfortably stretched on a bed or in an easy chair. Then try to relax your nerves, all together or one by one, till you have a complete relaxation. This done and while your body lies like a limp rag upon the bed, make your brain silent and immobile till it is no longer conscious of itself. Then slowly, imperceptibly pass from this state into sleep. When you will get up the next morning you will be full of energy. On the contrary, if you go to bed quite tired and without re-laxing .yourself, you will drop into a heavy, dense and uncon-scious sleep in which the vital will lose all its energies.

It is possible you may not obtain an immediate result, but persevere.

Relax the Whole Mind

There are countless dreams without any connection which have no interest. For your brain is like a recording instrument: something comes and strikes hundreds of cells, each thing must strike a small note. Things will strike the brain con-volutions — a remembrance, an impression, all kinds of tiny memories — it depends on your condition. But you have the control, ideas follow each other in accordance with a certain logic; there is also a mechanism which puts memories into movement through contagion, and the movement through contagion is made according to logic (what you call logic). But when you sleep, that faculty usually goes to sleep, so all those little cells are left to themselves and the connections — like the connections of electric wires — don't work any longer, things come the wrong way round or in any direction at all. You must not look for a meaning. It was a contagion: because this one was vibrating, that other also vibrated, one vibration gives rise to another. Your logic works no longer. And you have fantastic dreams, absurd dreams.

It is very difficult to put one's mind into repose. The major-ity of men get up very tired, more tired than when they went to sleep. One must learn how to quieten one's mind, make it completely blank, and then when one wakes up, one feels refreshed. One must relax the whole mind in the pure white silence, then one has the least number of dreams.

22 April 1953

Relax, Give Yourself Up

How can one remain conscious in the midst of unconsciousness?

One must be vigilant.

And when asleep?

One can remain conscious in sleep, we have already explained that! One must work.

Then one doesn't sleep!

Not at all, one sleeps much better, one has a quiet sleep instead of a restless one. Most people do so many things in their sleep that they wake up more tired than before. We have already spoken about this once. Naturally, if you keep yourself from sleeping, you won't sleep. I always tell those who complain of not being able to sleep, "Meditate then and you will end up by sleeping." It is better to fall asleep while concentrating than "like that", scattered and strewn without knowing even where one is.

To sleep well one must learn how to sleep.

If one is physically very tired, it is better not to go to sleep immediately, otherwise one falls into the inconscient. If one is very tired, one must stretch out on the bed, relax, loosen all the nerves one after another until one becomes like a rumpled cloth in one's bed, as though one had neither bones nor muscles. When one has done that, the same thing must be done in the mind. Relax, do not concentrate on any idea or try to solve a problem or ruminate on impressions, sensations or emotions you had during the day. All that must be allowed to drop off quietly: one gives oneself up, one is indeed like a rag. When you have succeeded in doing this, there is always a little flame, there — that flame never goes out and you become conscious of it when you have managed this relaxation. And all of a sudden this little flame rises slowly into an aspiration for the divine life, the truth, the consciousness of the Divine, the union with the inner being, it goes higher and higher, it rises, rises, like that, very gently. Then everything gathers there, and if at that moment you fall asleep, you have the best sleep you could possibly have. I guarantee that if you do this carefully, you are sure to sleep, and also sure that instead of falling into a dark hole you will sleep in light, and when you get up in the morning you will be fresh, fit, content, happy and full of energy for the day.

When one is conscious in sleep, does the brain sleep or not?

When does the brain ever sleep? When does it sleep? This is of all things the most difficult. If you succeed in making your brain sleep, it would be wonderful. How it runs on! That is vagabondage. It is this I meant when I spoke of relaxation in the brain. If you do it really well, your brain enters a silent restfulness and that is wonderful; when you attain that, five minutes of that and you are quite fresh afterwards, you can solve a heap of problems.

If the brain is always working, why don't we remember what has happened during the night?

Because you have not caught the consciousness at its work. And perhaps because if you remembered what was going on in your brain, you would be horrified! It is really like a madhouse, all these ideas that clash, all dancing a saraband in the head! it is as if one were throwing balls in all directions at once. So, if you saw that, you would be a bit troubled.

23 April 1951

Rest in the State of Sachchidananda

Has the mind need of rest apart from the physical body and the physical brain?

Yes, an absolute need. And it is only in silence that the mind can receive the true light from above. I do not think that the mental being is liable to fatigue; if it feels tired, that is rather a reaction of the brain. It is only in silence that it can rise above itself. But from the point of view of sleep and dreams of which we were speaking, there is a very remarkable phenomenon. I have tried it out. If you are able to establish not only silence in your head but also repose in your vital, the stoppage of all the activities of your being, and if coming out of the domain of forms you enter into what is called Sachchidananda, the supreme consciousness, then with three minutes of that state you can have more rest than in eight hours of sleep. It is not very easy, no.... It is the consciousness absolutely conscious but completely still, in the full original Light. If you get that, if you are able to immobilise everything in you, then your whole being participates in this supreme consciousness and I have well observed that as regards rest (and I mean by rest bodily rest, the repose of the muscles) three minutes of that state were equivalent to eight hours of ordinary sleep.

27 January 1951

Dreamless Sleep

What is the nature of dreamless sleep?

Generally, when you have what you call dreamless sleep, it is one of two things; either you do not remember what you dreamt or you fell into absolute unconsciousness which is almost death — a taste of death. But there is the possibility of a sleep in which you enter into an absolute silence, immobility and peace in all parts of your being and your consciousness merges into Sachchidananda. You can hardly call it sleep, for it is extremely conscious. In that condition you may remain for a few minutes, but these few minutes give you more rest and refreshment than hours of ordinary sleep. You cannot have it by chance; it requires a long training.

21 April 1929

The Supreme Rest

Mother, you said that the sleep before midnight gives us most rest...

Physically, yes.

Why?

Ah! I said that through personal experience and then that...
There's no why about it, is there? Everyone should find this
out for himself, or not find it out. But I have heard from
those who are interested in earth-chemistry that there are
certain rays — (*turning to Pavitra*) isn't that so? Tell us, do
you know about it? — sun-rays which remain active in the
atmosphere till midnight, and other rays which become active
afterwards, and these give you strength and those draw it out
of you. But there are many things like that; at least this, you
understand, is something we hear of or read in books. I am
giving it to you for what it is worth. I know nothing. Somebody who is very well up in the subject could give you a fuller
explanation. (*Laughing*) But certain things are true, in practice. I cannot say why; perhaps they are only personal things!
But still, I have heard of a similar experience from others also.
For instance, you go into the sea, remain there a few minutes
and you come out full of strength. You go into the sea and remain in it for an hour and you come out completely exhausted!
Even with a hot bath it is the same thing. You have a hot bath;
you are very tired; you get into it; you remain there at the most
for a moment; you come out and feel quite fresh. You remain
there for a quarter of an hour, you come out, you have lost
all your strength, your energy, there's nothing left, you are
drained out.

I tell you this, I cannot speak to you with any competence
about the reason, but the fact is there. It is like that. For myself I have an explanation, but it is good only for me, it does
not work for others. So it is useless.

As for these stages of sleep which are spoken about here, if
one is conscious of one's nights, one can cover them in a few
minutes. One does not need to wait for hours of sleep to do
this, you understand; if one is conscious, one can pass through
all that in a few minutes. To begin with, when one is conscious

of one's nights, the first thing to do before falling fast asleep, just in the state when one begins to relax, relax all one's nerves — I have explained this to you already, one relaxes all the nerves and lets oneself go... like this... you know — well, at that moment, one must relax very carefully all mental activity and make that quiet, as quiet as possible, and not go off to sleep until the mind is quite calm. Then you escape quite a long period of useless excitement which is extremely tiring. If you can so manage that the mind relaxes and enters into a complete peace first, your sleep will immediately become very peaceful and very refreshing; naturally, your vital must not be in a turmoil, for then, in that case, it will take you into all sorts of places and make you commit all kinds of stupidities, and the result will be that you will wake up even more tired than when you went to sleep.

But if you are conscious, after having calmed your vital, when you begin to come out from your physical consciousness and enter a more subtle consciousness, you put your vital to sleep, you say to it, "Rest now, keep very quiet," and then you enter your mental activity and say to the mind, "Rest now, remain very quiet", and you put it to sleep also; and then you come out of the mind into a higher region, and there, if it begins to interest you, for instance, if it is the first time you have gone there, you may look at what is happening, have your experience, learn things — at times one learns very interesting things; and then, sometimes one can become aware of a certain general state also, have ideas about other people, other things; it is interesting! And later, if you have had enough of this, you say, "Keep quiet, sleep, don't move", and you put that to sleep, and rise to a still higher consciousness, and so on, till you reach a state where you are on the borders of *form*, I am not speaking of physical form — on the borders of all form, much higher than the form of thought, naturally; on the borders of all form and all vibration, in the perfect silence, what here we call Sachchidananda. And when you are there, everything stops, all vibrations subside, and if you remain there just three minutes, you come back to your body *absolutely* rested, refreshed, fortified, as though you had slept for hours! This is something one can learn to do. I don't say it can be done overnight, a little work is necessary and also some persistence, but still... this one must learn to do; and when you are very anxious, very tired, very... For instance, when you have just undergone violent attacks from hostile forces in one form or another, and are very tired, if you follow this process consciously, well, within a few minutes all that disappears completely. It is something worth learning. Only, one must be very, very, very persevering, for... Wait a bit, I am going to tell you something more about it.

When I began studying occultism, I became aware that — just when I began to work upon my nights in order to make them conscious — I became aware that there was between the subtle-physical and the most material vital a small region, very small, which was not sufficiently developed to serve as a conscious link between the two activities. So what took place in the consciousness of the most material vital did not get translated exactly in the consciousness of the most subtle-physical. Some of it got lost on the way because it was like a — not-positively a void but something only half-conscious, not sufficiently developed. I knew there was only one way, that was to work to develop it. I began working. This happened sometime about the month of February, I believe. One month, two months, three, four, no result. We go on. Five months, six months... it was at the end of July or the beginning of August. I left Paris, the house I was staying in, and went to the countryside, quite a small place on the seashore, to stay with some friends who had a garden. Now, in that garden there was a lawn — you know what a lawn is, don't you? grass — where there were flowers and around it some trees. It was a fine place, very quiet, very silent. I lay on the grass, like this, flat on my stomach, my elbows in the grass, and then suddenly all the life of that Nature, all the life of that region between the subtle-physical and the most material vital, which is very living in plants and in Nature, all that region became all at once, suddenly, without any transition, absolutely living, intense, conscious, marvellous; and this was the result, wasn't it? of six months of work which had given nothing. I had not noticed anything; but just a little condition like that and the result was there! It is like the chick in the egg, yes! It is there for a very long time and yet one sees nothing at all. And one wonders whether there is indeed a chick in the egg; and then, suddenly "Tick!", there is a tiny hole, you know, and then everything bursts and out comes the chick! It is quite ready, but it took all that time to be formed; that's how it is. When you want to prepare something within you, that is how it is, it is like the chick in the egg. You need a very long time, and this without having the least result, never getting discouraged, and continuing your effort, absolutely regularly, as though you had eternity before you and, moreover, as though you were quite disinterested about the result. You do the work because you do it. And then, suddenly, one day, it bursts and you see before you the full result of your work.

But you understand, don't you? one speaks like this, very easily, of becoming conscious of one's nights, having control over one's sleep-activities and all sorts of things of this kind, but you need to do many such little works like the one I have just described to you. Many of these are needed to obtain this result. When one is accomplished, you realise that there is another missing, and when this is done, you realise there is still another, and so on, until one fine day you can do what I said, and you go from one plane to another, like that, putting all to rest, until you come out of all activity and enter the supreme rest, consciously. It is worth the trouble.

23 June 1954

Nightmares and Digestion

If one eats a heavy meal, why is the sleep disturbed by nightmares?

Because there is a very close connection between dreams and the condition of the stomach. Observations have been made and it has been noticed that in accordance with what is eaten, dreams are of one kind or another, and that if the digestion is difficult, the dream always turns into a nightmare — those nightmares which have no reality but still are nightmares all the same and very unpleasant — seeing tigers, cats, etc.... Or else you experience things like... for instance, you are facing a great danger and must hurry up, get dressed quickly and go out, and then you can't dress, try as you will, you can't put on your things, you don't find your things any more, and if you want to put on your shoes they never fit you, and if you want to go somewhere very fast, the legs don't move any longer, they are paralysed and you are stuck there making formidable efforts to advance, and you can't move. It is this kind of nightmare that comes from a disordered stomach.

24 March 1954

Vital and Mental Nightmares

In vital nightmares, which part of the being goes out of the body?

Your vital — not the whole of it, for that would produce a cataleptic state, but a portion of the vital goes out for a stroll. Some always go to the nastiest places and so have very bad nights — the possibilities in these nightly rambles are innumerable. It may be a very small thing, just a little portion of your being, but if it is conscious, that is enough to give you a fine little nightmare!

You know, when you sleep, the inner beings are not concentrated upon the body, they go out and become more or less independent — a limited independence, but independence all the same — and they go to dwell in their own domains. The mind more so, for it is hardly held within the body, it is only concentrated but not contained in the body. The vital also goes beyond the body, but it is more concentrated upon the body. . . .

What is a "mental nightmare"?

When there is a chaos in the brain or a local fever, a particular turmoil in the brain, a brain-fag, or if there is a want of control, you let yourself be possessed by mental formations, this is what happens most often — mental formations which, most often, you yourself have made, besides. And as the control of the rational, waking consciousness has gone, all this begins to dance a saraband in the head, with a kind of raging madness; ideas get entangled, collide, fight, it is truly hallucinating. Then, unless you have the power to bring a great peace into your head, a great tranquillity, a very strong and pure light, well, it is ten times worse than a vital nightmare. The worst of a vital nightmare consists generally in fighting with an enemy who wants to kill you, and you strike him terrible blows, and the blows never hit; you exert all your force, all your energy, and you do not succeed in touching your adversary. He is there in front of you, he threatens you, he is going to strangle you and you gather all your strength, you try to strike, but nothing touches him. When the struggle is like that, hand to hand, with a being who throws himself upon you, it is particularly painful. That is why you are advised not to go out of the body unless you have the necessary power or the purity. You see, in this kind of nightmare the force you want to use is the "memory" of a physical force; but one may have great physical strength, be a first-class boxer, and yet be completely powerless in the vital world because one does not have the necessary vital power. As for the mental nightmare, that kind of frightful saraband in the head, one has altogether the impression of going mad.

10 March 1951

One Can Arrange One's Dreams

Sweet Mother, you have said that one can exercise one's conscious will and change the course of one's dreams.

Ah, yes, I have already told you that once. If you are in the middle of a dream and something happens which you don't like (for instance, somebody shouts that he wants to kill you), you say: "That won't do at all, I don't want my dream to be like that", and you can change the action or the ending. You can organise your dream as you want. One can arrange one's dreams. But for this you must be conscious that you are dreaming, you must know you are dreaming.

But these dreams are not of much importance, are they?

Yes, they are, and one must be conscious of what can happen. Suppose that you have gone for a stroll in the vital world; there you meet beings who attack you (that's what happens usually), if you know that it is a dream, you can very easily gather your vital forces and conquer. That's a true fact; you can with a certain attitude, a certain word, a certain way of being do things you would not do if you were just dreaming.

If in the dream someone kills you it doesn't matter, for it is just a dream!

I beg your pardon! Usually, the next day you are ill, or maybe a little later. That's a warning. I know someone whose eye was thus hurt in a dream, and who really lost his eye a few days later. As for me, once I happened to dream getting blows on my face. Well, when I woke up the next morning, I had a red mark in the same place, on the forehead and the cheek.... Inevitably, a wound received in the vital being is translated in the physical body.

But how does it happen? There must be some intermediary?

It was in the vital that I was beaten. It is from within that this comes. Nothing, nobody touched anything from outside. If you receive a blow in the vital, the body suffers the consequence. More than half of our illnesses are the result of blows of this kind, and this happens much oftener than one believes. Only, men are not conscious of their vital, and as they are not conscious they don't know that fifty per cent of their illnesses are the result of what happens in the vital: shocks, accidents, fighting, ill-will.... Externally this is translated by an illness. If one knows how it reacts on the physical, one goes to its source and can cure oneself in a few hours.

29 April 1953

Going Out of the Body and Somnambulism

Who among you has had the experience of going out of the body — going out and knowing about it? I do not even speak of doing it at will, for that is another stage.

Once I went out of my body but got back into it imme-
diately!

You did not take the opportunity of going for a little walk, did you? Well, you are not inquisitive!

How can one know that one has gone out of the body?

You see it immobile on your bed. There are other means of knowing also....

At times when one goes out of the body, the body follows
the part which goes out.

You are speaking of a somnambulist? But that is quite another thing. This means that the part which goes out (whether a part of the mind or a part of the vital) is so strongly attached to the body, or rather that the body is so attached to this part, that when this part decides to do something the body follows it automatically. In your inner being you decide to do a certain thing and your body is so closely tied to your inner being that without thinking of it, without wanting to do so, without making any effort, it follows and does the same thing. Note that in this matter, the physical body has capacities it would not have in the ordinary waking condition. For instance, it is well known that one can walk in dangerous places where one would find it rather difficult to walk in the waking state. The body follows the consciousness of the inner being and its own consciousness is asleep — for the body has a consiousness. All the parts of the being, including the most material, have an independent consciousness. Hence when you go to sleep dead tired, when your physical body needs rest absolutely, your physical consciousness sleeps, while the consciousness of your subtle physical body or your vital or of your mind does not sleep, it continues its activity; but your physical consciousness is separated from the body, it is asleep in a state of unconsciousness, and then the part which does not sleep, which is active, uses the body without the physical consciousness as intermediary and makes it do things directly. That is how one becomes a somnambulist. According to my experience, the waking consciousness goes to sleep, for some reason or other (usually due to fatigue), but the inner being is awake, and the body is so tied to it that it follows it automatically. That is why you do fantastic things, because you do not see them physically, you see them in a different way.

It is said that somnambulism is due to serious preoccupations and cares. Is this true? Tartini composed a sonata in this state, and when he got up in the morning, he wrote down the whole thing.

Somnambulism is not always due to preoccupations and cares! Yes, there are people who write wonderful things

when in somnambulism. But Tartini was not a somnambulist—
it was in the dream-state that he wrote sonatas.

The other state is always a little dangerous, always. Unexpected things can happen, an accident to the vital, for instance.

How can one be cured of somnambulism?

Quite simply, by putting a will upon the body before going to sleep. One becomes a somnambulist because the mind is not developed enough to break the inner ties. For the mind always separates the external being from the deeper consciousness. Little children are quite tied up. I knew children who were quite sincere but could not distinguish whether a thing was going on in their imagination or in reality. For them the inner life was as real as the external life. They were not telling stories, they were not liars; simply the inner life was as real as the external life. There are children who go night after night to the same spot in order to continue the dream they have begun — they are experts in the art of going out of their bodies.

Is it good to leave the body asleep and go out rambling?
Can one go back into the body at any moment one likes?

It is dangerous if you sleep surrounded by people who may come and shake you up, believing that something has happened to you. But if you are alone and sleep quietly, there is no danger.

One can get back into the body at any time and generally it is much more difficult to remain outside than to get back — as soon as the least thing happens, one rushes back quickly into the body. . . .

People who have nightmares . . . should always protect themselves occultly before going out of the body — it can be done in many ways. The simplest way, one which needs no special knowledge is to call the Guru or, if one knows somebody who has the knowledge, to call him in thought or spirit; or to protect oneself by making a kind of wall of protection around oneself (one can do many things, can't one?)....

If you have a disposition for exteriorisation and if you follow a yoga, you are always asked to protect your sleep: by some contemplation, a mental movement, any movement — there are many ways of protecting oneself.

19 February 1951

3

FOOD AND DRINK

Eat for Living

Eat for living but do not live for eating.

*

Greed for anything concerning physical consciousness, so-called necessities and comfort of whatever nature — this is one of the most serious obstacles to sadhana.

Each little satisfaction you get through greed is one step backward from the goal.

*

A sadhak must eat because of his body's need of hunger and not because of the demands of his greed.

*

When you have a desire you are governed by the thing you desire, it takes possession of your mind and your life, and you become a slave. If you have greed for food you are no more the master of food, it is the food that masters you.

*

Unless you control the food you take, you will always be ill.

*

It is an inner attitude of freedom from attachment and from greed of food and desire of the palate that is needed, not undue diminution of the quantity taken or any self-starvation. One must take sufficient food for the maintenance of the body and its strength and health but without attachment or desire.

*

One thing we want to know is how much you are eating and whether you sleep regularly and sufficiently. These two points are of great importance, for a sadhana of this kind demands in order to bear it that the mind and body and nervous system should not be weakened by undernourishment and lack of sleep.

*

It is not by fasting but by improving the will that one obtains the Truth.

*

In the effect of food on the body, 90% belongs to the power of thought.

*

In fact I can assure you that the pain in the stomach as well as many other discomforts are due 90% to wrong thinking and strong imaginations — I mean that the material basis for them is practically negligible.

Indifference towards Food

The ordinary life is a round of various desires and greeds. As long as one is preoccupied with them, there can be no lasting progress. A way out of the round must be discovered. Take, as an instance, that commonest preoccupation of ordinary life — the constant thinking by people of what they will eat and when they will eat and whether they are eating enough. To conquer the greed for food an equanimity in the being must be developed such that you are perfectly indifferent towards food. If food is given you, you eat it; if not, it does not worry you in the least; above all, you do not keep thinking about food. And the thinking must not be negative, either. To be absorbed in devising methods and means of abstinence as the *sannyasis* do is to be almost as preoccupied with food as to be absorbed in dreaming of it greedily. Have an attitude of indifference towards it: that is the main thing. Get the idea of food out of your consciousness, do not attach the slightest importance to it.

1930-1931

Preference for Food

And then, finally, habits!... There is a charming phrase here — I appreciated it fully — in which Sri Aurobindo is asked, "What is meant by 'the physical adhering to its own habits'?" What are the habits of the physical which it must throw off? It is this *terrible, frightful* preference for the food you were used to when you were very young, the food you ate in the country where you were born and about which you feel when you no longer get it that you have not anything at all to eat, that you are miserable!

I don't know, I believe there wouldn't be a dozen people here who have come to the Ashram and eaten the food of the Ashram without saying, "Oh! I am not used to this food. It is very difficult." And how many, how many hundreds of people who prepare their own food because they cannot eat the food of the Ashram! (*Mother slams the book down on the stool, then continues to speak*): And then, they justify this! So it is here that these ideas begin to come, and they say, "My health! I can't digest well!" All this is only in their head. There is not a word of truth in it. NOT ONE WORD OF TRUTH. It is a perpetual lie in which everybody lives, and in this matter, indeed, I may tell you what I think, you have not advanced any farther than the mass of human beings!

I make an exception for the very, very, very rare ones who are not like that. They could be counted on one's fingers. And all, all justify this, all, all — "Oh, my poor children! They are not used to eating this food. How shall we manage? They will die because of this change of food!" Well, I, indeed, can give a remedy for that. You take a boat, take a train and go round the world several times, you are obliged to eat in each country the food of that country, and after you have done this several times, you will understand your stupidity!... It is a stupidity. A frightful *tamas*! One is tied up there like this (*Mother makes a movement with her hands*) to one's gastric habits!

9 June 1954

Food: The Old Habits

Mother, the Ashram has been here for a long time; and you say the people who have done something could be counted on your fingers...

No, no, I didn't say that. (*Laughter*) I was speaking only of food. I was speaking of those who came here and who did not begin, you understand, who did not... The story is very interesting. There are people who come, full of goodwill, moreover — I think I have written this somewhere in the *Bulletin* — their goodwill is so overflowing that when they arrive everything is perfect, including the food. They find it very good as long as they are in their psychic consciousness. When *that* begins to go down, the old habits begin to rise up; you understand, when the psychic consciousness comes down, the old habits climb back into their place. And then they begin saying: "It is strange! I used to like this, but I don't like it any more; it has become bad, this food!" This is an intermediary period, and later, after sometime, more or less shyly according to their nature they say (*Mother begins whispering*), "Couldn't I have my personal food? For... I don't know, my stomach does not digest this!" (*Laughter*) Well, I say that among the people in the Ashram, I am not sure... but there are very, very few who haven't done that. And those who have told themselves: "Oh, as for me, it is all the same to me, I eat what I am given, and I don't bother about it" — these, indeed, can truly be counted on your fingers.

One must look at the thing very clearly, you understand, for there are some who do not dare to speak, many do not dare to say anything, except when they are a little indisposed or really have a stomach-ache or they think they have a stomach-ache and go to see a doctor. The doctor tells them, "Oh, try this or try that and see" — just the things they were accustomed to eating. The doctor begins by asking them, "What were you used to eating formerly?" (*Laughter*) "Weren't you used to taking this?" (*Laughter*) In this way. Then naturally, immediately they say, "Yes, yes, yes, I think that will do me good!" (*Laughter*)

9 June 1954

Regarding Attachment to Food

Now, if it so happens that you have decided to progress and if you enter the path of yoga, then a new factor intervenes. As soon as you want to progress, you immediately meet the resistance of everything that does not want to progress both in you and around you. And this resistance naturally expresses itself in all the thoughts that correspond to it.

Suppose that you want to make a progress regarding attachment to food, for example; well, almost constantly there will come to you thoughts particularly interested in food, about what should be taken, what should not be taken, how it should be taken, how it should not be taken; and these ideas will come to you, they will seem quite natural to you. And the more you say within yourself, "Oh! how I would like to be free from all that, what a hindrance to my progress are all these preoccupations", the more will they come, quietly, until the progress is truly made within and you have risen to a level of consciousness where you can see all these things from above and put them *in their place* — which is not a very big place in the universe! And so on, for all things. Therefore, your occupations and affinities are going to put you almost contradictorily into contact not only with ideas having an affinity and relation with your way of being, but with the opposite. And if you don't take care from the beginning to keep an attitude of discernment, you will be turned into a mental battlefield.

If you know how to rise to a higher level, simply into a region of the speculative mind which is not quite the ordinary physical mind, you can see all this play and all this struggle, all this conflict, all these contradictions as a curiosity which does not touch or affect you. If you rise a step higher still and see the goal towards which you want to go, you will gradually come to discern between ideas favourable to your progress which you will keep, and ideas opposed to this progress which harm and impair it; and from above you will have the power to set them aside, calmly, without being otherwise affected by them. But if you remain there, at that level in the midst of that confusion and conflict, well, you risk getting a headache!

The best thing to do is to occupy yourself with something practical which will compel you to concentrate specially: studies, work or some physical occupation for the body which demands attention — anything at all that forces you to concentrate on what you are doing and no longer be a prey to these ramblings. But if you have the misfortune to remain there and look at them, then surely, as I said, you will get a headache. For it is a problem which must be resolved either by a descent into practical life and a concentration on some practical effort or else by rising above and looking from above at all this chaos so as to be able to bring some order into it and set it right.

But one must never remain on the same plane, it is a plane which is no good either for physical or moral health.

27 June 1956

The So-called Needs of the Body

Sri Aurobindo speaks [in *The Synthesis of Yoga*] of physical needs, the needs of the body, which are generally considered as imperative and which have their own truth; he says that even that can be only quite a partial light, that is to say, a semblance of knowledge or even something false.

That goes against all modern ideas.

People always have the impression that what they call the needs of the body, what the body demands, is an absolute law;

that if it is not obeyed, well, one commits a great wrong against one's body which will suffer the consequences. And Sri Aurobindo says that these needs in themselves are either very partial lights, that is to say, only a way of seeing things, or even no lights at all — completely false.

If one were to study the problem attentively enough, one would find out to what an extent these so-called needs of the body depend on the mental attitude. For example, the need to eat. There are people who literally die of hunger if they have not eaten for eight days. There are others who do it deliberately and observe fasting as a principle of yoga, as a necessity in yoga. And for them, at the end of eight days' fasting, the body is as healthy as when they started, and sometimes healthier!

Finally, for all these things, it is a question of proportion, of measure. It is obvious that one can't always live without eating. But it is as obvious that the idea people have about the need to eat is not true. Indeed, it is a whole subject for study: the importance of the mental attitude in relation to the body.

Sri Aurobindo does not recognise the needs of the body as things true in themselves. He says: it is not true, it is only an idea you have, an impression, it is not something true which carries its truth in itself.

16 May 1956

Freedom Even from All Need for Food

It is not by abstaining from food that you can make a spiritual progress. It is by being free, not only from all attachment and all desire and preoccupation with food, but even from all need for it; by being in the state in which all these things are so foreign to your consciousness that they have no place there.

Only then, as a spontaneous, natural result, can one usefully stop eating. It could be said that the essential condition is to forget to eat — forget, because all the energies of the being and all its concentration are turned towards a more total, more true inner realisation, towards this *constant*, imperative pre-occupation with the union of the whole being, including the bodily cells, with the vibration of the divine forces, with the supramental force which is manifesting, so that this may be the true life: not only the purpose of life, but the essence of life, not only an imperative need of life, but all its joy and all its *raison d'être*.

When that is there, when this realisation is attained, then to eat or not to eat, to sleep or not to sleep, all this has no longer any importance. It is an outer rhythm left to the play of the universal forces as a whole, finding expression through the circumstances and people around you; and the body, united, totally united with the inner truth, has a suppleness, a constant adaptability: if food is there, it takes it; if it isn't there, it doesn't think about it....

12 June 1957

If One Eats Meat

"*Is taking very little food helpful in controlling the senses?*"

"*No. It simply exasperates them — to take a moderate amount is best. People who fast easily get exalted and may lose their balance.*"

"*If one takes only vegetarian food, does it help in controlling the senses?*"

"*It avoids some of the difficulties which the meat-eaters have, but it is not sufficient by itself.*"

Sri Aurobindo, Elements of Yoga

Any questions?

What happens if one eats meat?

Do you want me to tell you a story? I knew a lady, a young Swedish woman, who was doing sadhana; and she was by habit a vegetarian, from both choice and habit. One day she was invited by some friends who gave her chicken for dinner. She did not want to make a fuss, she ate the chicken. But afterwards, during the night suddenly she found herself in a basket with her head between two pieces of wicker-work, shaken, shaken, shaken, and feeling wretched, miserable; and then, after that she found herself head down, feet in the air, and being shaken, shaken, shaken. (*Laughter*) She felt perfectly miserable; and then all of a sudden, somebody began pulling out things from her body, and that hurt her terribly, and then someone came along with a knife and chopped off her head; and then she woke up. She told me all this; she said she had never had such a frightful nightmare, that she had not thought of anything before going to sleep, that it was just the consciousness of the poor chicken that had entered her, and that she had experienced in her dream all the anguish the poor chicken had suffered when it was carried to the market, sold, its feathers plucked and its neck cut! (*Laughter*)

That's what happens! That is to say, in a greater or lesser proportion you swallow along with the meat a little of the consciousness of the animal you eat. It is not very serious, but it is not always very pleasant. And obviously it does not help you in being on the side of man rather than of the beast! It is evident that primitive men, those who were still much closer to the beast than the spirit, apparently used to eat raw meat, and that gives much more strength than cooked meat. They killed the animal, tore it apart and bit into it, and they were very strong. And moreover, this is why there was in their intestines that little piece, the appendix which in those days was much bigger and served to digest the raw meat. And then man began to cook. He found out that things tasted better that way, and he ate cooked meat and gradually the appendix grew smaller and was no longer of any use at all. So now it is an encumbrance which at times brings on an illness.

This is to tell you that perhaps now it is time to change one's food and go over to something a little less bestial! It depends absolutely on each one's state of consciousness. For an ordinary man, living an ordinary life, having ordinary activities, not thinking at all of anything else except earning his living, of keeping himself fit and perhaps taking care of his family, it is good to eat meat, it is all right for him to eat anything at all, whatever agrees with him, whatever does him good.

But if one wishes to pass from this ordinary life to a higher one, the problem begins to become interesting; and if, after having come to a higher life, one tries to prepare oneself for the transformation, then it becomes very important. For there certainly are foods which help the body to become subtle and others which keep it in a state of animality. But it is only at that particular time that this becomes very important, not before; and before reaching that moment, there are many other things to do. Certainly it is better to purify one's mind and purify one's vital before thinking of purifying one's body. For even if you take all possible precautions and live physically taking care not to absorb anything except what will help to subtilise your body, if your mind and vital remain in a state of desire, inconscience, darkness, passion and all the rest, that won't be of any use at all. Only, your body will become weak, dislocated from the inner life and one fine day it will fall ill.

One must begin from inside, I have already told you this once. One must begin from above, first purify the higher and then purify the lower. I am not saying that one must indulge in all sorts of degrading things in the body. That's not what I am telling you. Don't take it as an advice not to exercise control over your desires! It isn't that at all. But what I mean is, do not try to be an angel in the body if you are not already just a little of an angel in your mind and vital; for that would dislocate you in a different way from the usual one, but not one that is better. We said the other day that what is most important is to keep the equilibrium. Well, to keep the equilibrium everything must progress at the same time. You must not leave one part of your being in darkness and try to bring the other into light. You must take great care not to leave any corner dark. There you are.

Why were eggs forbidden in the Ashram formerly? Now you give eggs.

Eggs were forbidden?

I don't know. That's what we were told.

Ah, people say many things, but I am not responsible for all the things they say! (*Laughter*) I don't remember ever refusing an egg to someone who needed it from the point of view of health. But if people come and ask for something just out of greediness, for pleasure, I always refuse, as much now as before. It is only from the point of view of health, you know, of the physical equilibrium, that certain things are allowed. Everything is allowed. I haven't refused meat to one who needed it. There were people who ate it because they needed it. But if someone comes asking me for something just in order to satisfy a desire, I say "No," whatever it may be, even ice-cream! (*Laughter*)

When one eats an egg, doesn't one eat the chicken inside it?

It's not yet formed, the consciousness of the chicken. Of course, one must take care to eat the egg fresh before the chick begins to be formed.

Sweet Mother, if the agony of a chicken can attack us, so too can that of a beetroot or a carrot, can't it?

For all that, I believe the chicken is more conscious than the beetroot. (*Laughter*) But I ought to tell you my own experience. Only I was thinking this was not something common.

In Tokyo I had a garden and in this garden I was growing vegetables myself. I had a fairly big garden and many vegetables. And so, every morning I used to go for a walk, after having watered them and all the rest; I used to walk around to choose which vegetables I could take for eating. Well, just imagine! there were some which said to me, "No, no, no, no, no."... and then there were others which called, and I saw them from a distance, and they were saying, "Take me, take me, take me!" So it was very simple, I looked for those which wanted to be taken and never did I touch those which did not. I used to think it was something exceptional. I loved my plants very much, I used to look after them, I had put a lot of consciousness into them while watering them, cleaning them, so I thought they had a special capacity, perhaps.

But in France it was the same thing. I had a garden also in the south of France where I used to grow peas, radishes, carrots. Well, there were some which were happy, which asked to be taken and eaten, and there were those which said, "No, no, no, don't touch me, don't touch me!" (*Laughter*)

Why did they say that, Sweet Mother?

Well, I experimented precisely to find out; and the result was not always the same. At times it was indeed that the plant was not edible; it was not good, it was hard or bitter, it was not good for eating. At other times it happened that it was not ready, that it was too early; it wasn't ripe. By waiting for a day or two, a day or two later it said to me, "Take me, take me, take me!" (*Laughter*)

23 June 1954

The Food of Tomorrow

There will be an attempt to find the food of tomorrow. Well, all this labour for assimilation that makes you so heavy — it takes so much time and energy of the person — it ought to be done *before* and you must be given something which is at once capable of being assimilated, as is done now: for example, they have vitamins that are directly assimilable and also... proteins, the nutritious principles that are found in such and such things and that are not bulky — a huge quantity is required to assimilate just a little. So now that they are clever enough from the chemical point of view, one is able to simplify. People do not like it simply because... because they take an intense delight in eating, but when one does not take pleasure in eating, one requires nourishment and does not lose time in that. You lose time enormously: the time for eating, the time for digesting and all the rest.

30 December 1967

Consecrating One's Food to God

Physically, we depend upon food to live — unfortunately. For with food, we daily and constantly take in a formidable amount of inconscience, of *tamas*, heaviness, stupidity. One can't do otherwise — unless constantly, without a break, we remain completely aware and, as soon as an element is introduced into our body, we immediately work upon it to extract from it only the light and reject all that may darken our consciousness. This is the origin and rational explanation of the religious practice of consecrating one's food to God before taking it. When eating one aspires that this food may not be taken for the little human ego but as an offering to the divine consciousness within oneself. In all yogas, all religions, this is encouraged. This is the origin of that practice, of contacting the consciousness behind, precisely to diminish as much as possible the absorption of an inconscience which increases daily, constantly, without one's being aware of it.

19 April 1951

Tobacco and Alcohol

Why do tobacco and alcohol destroy the memory and will?

Why! Because they do so. There is no moral reason. It is a fact. There is a poison in alcohol, there is a poison in tobacco; and this poison goes into the cells and damages them. Alcohol is never expelled so to say, it accumulates in a certain part of the brain, and then, after the accumulation, these cells no longer function at all — some people, even go mad because of it, that is what is called *delirium tremens*, the result of having swallowed too much alcohol which is not absorbed but remains in this way concentrated in the brain. And it is so radical even that... There is a province in France, for instance, which produces wine, a wine with a very low percentage of alcohol: I believe it is four or five per cent, a very low percentage, you understand; and these people, because they make it, drink wine as one drinks water. They drink it neat, and after some time they become ill. They have cerebral disorders. I knew people of this kind, the brain was disordered, didn't function any more. And tobacco — nicotine is a very serious poison. It is a poison that destroys the cells. I have said that it is a slow poison because one doesn't feel it immediately except when one smokes for the first time and it makes one very ill. And this should make you understand that it ought not to be done. Only, people are so stupid that they think it is a weakness and so continue until they get used to the poison. And the body no longer reacts, it allows itself to be destroyed without reacting: you get rid of the reaction.

24 March 1954

4

SELF-CONTROL

In Life One Must Choose

In life, one must choose between a disordered and useless life of desires and that of an ascent into the light of aspiration and mastery of one's lower nature.

*

First learn to know yourself perfectly and then to control yourself perfectly. You will be able to do it by aspiring every moment. It is never too early to begin, never too late to continue.

*

There is no greater victory than that of controlling oneself.

*

Self-mastery is the greatest conquest, it is the basis of all enduring happiness.

*

To conquer a desire brings more joy than to satisfy it.

*

When one is incapable of conforming to a discipline, one is also incapable of doing anything of lasting value in life.

*

To discipline one's life is not easy, even for those who are strong, severe with themselves, courageous and enduring.

But before trying to discipline one's whole life, one must at least try to discipline *one* activity and persist until one succeeds.

Self-control

There are human beings. . . . who indulge in vice — one vice or another, like drinking or drug-injections — and who know very well that this is leading them to destruction and death. But they choose to do it, knowingly.

They have no control over themselves.

There is always a moment when everyone has self-control. And if one had not said "Yes" once, if one had not taken the decision, one would not have done it.

There is not one human being who has not the energy and capacity to resist something imposed upon him — if he is left free to do so. People tell you, "I can't do otherwise" — it is because in the depths of their heart they *do not want* to do otherwise; they have accepted to be the slaves of their vice. There is a moment when one accepts.

And I would go even further; I say, there is a moment when one accepts to be ill. If one did not accept to be ill, one would not be ill. Only, people are so unconscious of themselves and their inner movements that they are not even aware of what they do.

4 January 1956

Obeying the Reason

This is . . . one of the first things for which all physical training is useful: the fact that it cannot be done really well unless the body is in the habit of obeying the reason rather than the vital impulse. For instance, the whole development of bodily perfection, of physical culture with dumb-bells and the exercises which have nothing particularly exciting and demand a discipline, habits which must be regular, reasonable, which give no scope to passion, desire, impulse — one must order one's life according to a very strict and very regular discipline — well, in order to do them really well one must be in the habit of governing one's life by the reason.

This is not very common. Usually, unless one has taken good care to make it otherwise, the impulses — the impulses of desire — all the enthusiasms and passions with all their reactions are the masters of human life. One must already be something of a sage to be able to undergo a rigorous discipline of the body and obtain from it the ordered, regular effort which can perfect it. There is no longer any room there for all the fancies of desire. You see, as soon as one gives way to excesses, to immoderation of any kind and a disorderly life, it becomes quite impossible to control one's body and develop it normally, not to mention that, naturally, one spoils one's health and as a result the most important part of the ideal of a perfect body disappears; for with bad health, impaired health, one is not much good for anything. And it is certainly the satisfaction of desires and impulses of the vital or the unreasonable demands of certain ambitions which make the body suffer and fall ill.

Naturally, there is all the ignorance of those who don't even know the most elementary rules of life; but everybody knows one must learn how to live and, for instance, that fire burns and water can drown! People don't need to be told all that, it is something they learn fast as they grow up; but the fact that the control of reason over life is absolutely indispensable even for good health, is not always accepted by the inferior man for whom life has no savour unless he can live out his passions.

I remember a man who came here a very long time ago, to stand as a candidate for the government. It so happened that he was introduced to me because they wanted my opinion of him, and so he asked me questions about the Ashram and the life we lead here, and about what I considered to be an indispensable discipline for life. This man used to smoke the whole day and drank much more than was necessary, and so he complained, you see, that he was often tired and sometimes could not control himself. I told him, "You know, first of all, you must stop smoking and you must stop drinking." He looked at me with an unbelievable bewilderment and said, "But then, if one doesn't either smoke or drink, it is not worth living!" I told him, "If you are still at that stage, it is no use saying anything more." . . .

It is a good thing to begin to learn at an early age that to lead an efficient life and obtain from one's body the maximum it is able to give, reason must be the master of the house. And it is not a question of yoga or higher realisation, it is something which should be taught everywhere, in every school, every family, every home: man was made to be a mental being, and merely to be a man — we are not speaking of anything else, we are speaking only of being a man — life must be dominated by reason and not by vital impulses. This should be taught to all children from their infancy.

8 May 1957

5

PHYSICAL CULTURE

Become Master of Your Body

Become Master of your body — this will lead you to Freedom.

*

Build in yourself the total harmony, so that when the time comes Perfect Beauty can express itself through your body.

*

Physical culture is the best way of developing the consciousness of the body, and the more the body is conscious, the more it is capable of receiving the divine forces that are at work to transform it and give birth to the new race.

*

The physical being itself can be the seat of perfect existence, knowledge and bliss.

Follow a Physical Discipline

To be a leader one must master one's ego, and to master one's ego is the first indispensable step for doing yoga. And this is what can make sports a powerful aid for the realisation of the Divine.

Very few people understand this, and generally those who are against this outer discipline of sports, this concentration on the material realisation, are people who *completely* lack control over their physical being. And to realise the integral yoga of Sri Aurobindo the control of one's body is a first *indispensable* step. Those who despise physical activities are people who won't be able to take a single step on the true path of integral yoga, unless they first get rid of their contempt. Control of the body in all its forms is an indispensable basis. A body which dominates you is an enemy, it is a disorder you cannot accept. It is the enlightened will in the mind which should govern the body, and not the body which should impose its law on the mind. When one knows that a thing is bad, one must be capable of not doing it. When one wants something to be realised, one must be able to do it and not be stopped at every step by the body's inability or ill-will or lack of collaboration; and for that one must follow a physical discipline and become master in one's own home.

It is very fine to escape into meditation and from the height of one's so-called grandeur look down on material things, but one who is not master in his own home is a slave.

10 April 1957

To Bear the Pressure of the Divine Descent

The movement in the inner being may be perfect; but it puts you in a certain condition of receptivity to forces that fill you with intense emotional excitement, if your external being is weak or untransformed. Where the external being offers resistance to the inner being or cannot hold the entirety of the Ananda, there is this confusion and anarchy in expression.

You must have a strong body and strong nerves. You must have a strong basis of equanimity in your external being. If you have this basis, you can contain a world of emotion and yet not have to scream it out. This does not mean that you cannot express your emotion, but you can express it in a beautiful harmonious way. To weep or scream or dance about is always a proof of weakness, either of the vital or the mental or the physical nature. . . .

If you have to bear the pressure of the Divine Descent, you must be very strong and powerful, otherwise you would be shaken to pieces. Some persons ask, "Why has not the Divine come yet?" Because you are not ready. If a little drop makes you sing and dance and scream what would happen if the whole thing came down?

Therefore do we say to people who have not a strong and firm and capacious basis in the body and the vital and the mind, "Do not pull", meaning "Do not try to pull at the forces of the Divine, but wait in peace and calmness." For they would not be able to bear the descent. But to those who possess the necessary basis and foundation we say, on the contrary, "Aspire and draw." For they would be able to receive and yet not be upset by the forces descending from the Divine.

14 April 1929

Equanimity in the External Being

What is it that you call "the basis of equanimity in the external being"?

It is good health, a solid body, well poised; when one does not have the nerves of a little girl that are shaken by the least thing; when one sleeps well, eats well. . . . When one is quite calm, well balanced, very quiet, one has a solid basis and can receive a large number of forces.

If anyone among you has received spiritual forces, forces of the Divine, Ananda, for example, he knows from experience that unless he is in good health he cannot contain them, keep them. He begins to weep and cry, gets restless to expend what he has received. He must laugh and talk and gesticulate, otherwise he cannot keep them, he feels stifled. And so by laughing, weeping, moving about he throws out what he has received.

To be well balanced, to be able to absorb what one receives, one must be very quiet, very calm. One must have a solid basis, good health. One must have a very solid basis. That is very important.

15 April 1953

The Body: Obedience, Endurance, Beauty

"By means of a rational and discerning physical educa-tion, we must make our body strong and supple enough to become a fit instrument in the material world for the truth-force which wants to manifest through us.

"In fact, the body must not rule, it must obey. By its very nature it is a docile and faithful servant. Unfor-tunately, it rarely has the capacity of discernment it ought to have with regard to its masters, the mind and the vital. It obeys them blindly, at the cost of its own well-being. The mind with its dogmas, its rigid and arbitrary principles, the vital with its passions, its excesses and dissipations soon destroy the natural balance of the body and create in it fatigue, exhaustion and disease."

The Mother, The Science of Living

It is much easier to organise the body than the vital, for in-

stance. But the mind and the vital, with the character and temperament they have, what do they not do with this poor slave
of a body! After having ill-treated it, perhaps ruined it (it
protests a little, falls ill a little), this is what the two accomplices
say: "What a beast is this body, it cannot follow us in our
movements!" Unhappily, the body obeys its masters, the
mind and the vital, blindly, without any discrimination. The
mind comes along with its theories: "You must not eat that, it
will harm you, you must not do that, it is bad", and if the mind
is not wise and clear-sighted, the poor body suffers the consequences of the orders it receives. I do not speak of the orders
it receives from the vital. The mind with its rigid principles
and the vital with its excesses and outbursts and passions are
quick to destroy the body's equilibrium and to create a condition of fatigue, exhaustion and illness.

> "*It must be freed from this tyranny and this can be done
> only through a constant union with the psychic centre of
> the being.*"
>
> *Ibid.*

That is evidently the cure of all ills.

> "*The body has a wonderful capacity of adaptation and
> endurance. It is able to do so many more things than one
> usually imagines. If, instead of the ignorant and despotic
> masters that now govern it, it is ruled by the central truth
> of the being, you will be amazed at what it is capable of
> doing.*"
>
> *Ibid.*

During the last war, it was proved that the body was capable
of enduring such suffering as is normally impossible to endure.

You have surely read or heard these stories of war in which the body was made to suffer and endure terrible things, and it withstood all that, it proved that it had almost inexhaustible capacities of endurance. Some people happened to be under conditions that should have killed them; if they survived, it was because they had in them a very strong will to survive and the body obeyed that will.

> *"In this sound and balanced life a new harmony will manifest in the body, reflecting the harmony of the higher regions, which will give it perfect proportions and ideal beauty of form."*
>
> *Ibid.*

That is the last stage. If you compare the human body as it now is with a higher ideal of beauty, obviously very few would pass the examination. In almost everyone there is a sort of unbalance in the proportions; we are so accustomed to it that we do not notice it, but if we look from the standpoint of the higher beauty, it becomes visible; very few bodies would bear comparison with perfect beauty. There are a thousand reasons for this unbalance but only one remedy, to instil into the being this instinct, this sense of true beauty, a supreme beauty which will gradually act on the cells and make the body capable of expressing beauty. This is still a thing which is not known: the body is infinitely more plastic than you believe. . . .

You could get much more from your body if you only took the trouble.

You must not despise it nor scold it too much, for it is not the culprit; if you follow a suitable method to train and educate your body, you will have an infinitely greater output than you have now. It is quite recently that men have begun to speak of physical culture as an important thing; if you go back a hundred years, it was the privilege of those who had nothing else to do. A hundred years ago it was a luxury. When someone said, "I do not want to send my child to school, he must earn his living", there were many who answered, "No, pardon me, you make a serious mistake, if you do not prepare your child for his adult life, he will be incapable of doing what he should do." People said this about the mind but it was not said about the body. So many children lived in more or less good conditions, with a body which was indeed a difficulty, but it used to be said, "That will get corrected, that will be all right...." With training and patience you can acquire a body with which you can get along in life. Nowadays, people recognise the value of a healthy and balanced life.

25 January 1951

What Is Physical Culture?

If we cultivate the body by a clear-sighted and rational method, at the same time we are helping the growth of the soul, its progress and enlightenment.

Physical culture is the process of infusing consciousness into the cells of the body. One may or may not know it, but it is a fact. When we concentrate to make our muscles move according to our will, when we endeavour to make our limbs more supple, to give them an agility, or a force, or a resistance, or a plasticity which they do not naturally possess, we infuse into the cells of the body a consciousness which was not there before, thus turning it into an increasingly homogeneous and receptive instrument, which progresses in and by its activities. This is the primary importance of physical culture. Of course, that is not the only thing that brings consciousness into the body, but it is something which acts in an overall way, and this is rare. I have already told you several times that the artist infuses a very great consciousness into his hands, as the intellectual does into his brain. But these are, as it were, local phenomena, whereas the action of physical culture is more general. And when one sees the absolutely marvellous results of this culture, when one observes the extent to which the body is capable of perfecting itself, one understands how useful this can be to the action of the psychic being which has entered into this material substance. For naturally, when it is in possession of an organised and harmonised instrument which is full of strength and suppleness and possibilities, its task is greatly facilitated.

I do not say that people who practise physical culture necessarily do it for this purpose, because very few are aware of this result. But whether they are aware of it or not, this is the result. Moreover, if you are at all sensitive, when you observe the moving body of a person who has practised physical culture in a methodical and rational way, you see a light, a consciousness, a life, which is not there in others.

There are always people with a wholly external view of things who say, "Workers, for example, who have to do hard physical labour and who are compelled by their work to learn to carry heavy weights — they too build up their muscles, and instead of spending their time like aristocrats doing exercises with no useful outward results, they at least produce something." This is ignorance. Because there is an essential difference between the muscles developed through specialised, local and limited use and muscles which have been cultivated deliberately and harmoniously according to an integral programme which leaves no part of the body without work or exercise.

People like workers and peasants, who have a specialised

occupation and develop only certain muscles, always end up with occupational deformities. And this in no way helps their psychic progress because, although the whole of life necessarily contributes to the psychic development, it does so in such an unconscious way and so slowly that the poor psychic being must come back again and again and again, indefinitely, to achieve its purpose. Therefore we can say without fear of being mistaken that physical culture is the sadhana of the body and that all sadhana necessarily helps to hasten the achievement of the goal. The more consciously you do it, the quicker and more general the result, but even if you do it blindly, if you can see no further than the tips of your fingers or your feet or your nose, you help the overall development.

Finally, one can say that any discipline that is followed rigorously, sincerely, deliberately, is a considerable help, for it enables life on earth to attain its goal more rapidly and prepares it to receive the new life. To discipline oneself is to hasten the arrival of this new life and the contact with the supramental reality.

As it is, the physical body is truly nothing but a very disfigured shadow of the eternal life of the Self. But this physical body is capable of progressive development; through each individual formation, the physical substance progresses, and one day it will be capable of building a bridge between physical life as we know it and the supramental life which is to manifest.

28 November 1958

Conscious Will

How is it that the movements we make almost constantly in our everyday life, or which we have to make in our work if it is a physical work, do not help or help very little, almost negligibly, to develop the muscles and to create harmony in the body? These same movements, on the other hand, if they are made consciously, deliberately, with a definite aim, suddenly start helping you to form your muscles and build up your body. There are jobs, for instance, where people have to carry extremely heavy loads, like bags of cement or sacks of corn or coal, and they make a considerable effort; to a certain extent they do it with an acquired facility, but that doesn't give them harmony of the body, because they don't do it with the *idea* of developing their muscles, they do it just "like that". And someone who follows a method, either one he has learnt or one he has worked out for himself, and who makes these very movements with the will to develop this muscle or that, to create a general harmony in his body — he succeeds. Therefore, in the conscious will, there is something which adds considerably to the movement itself. Those who really want to practise physical culture as it is conceived now, everything they do, they do consciously. They walk downstairs consciously, they make the movements of ordinary life consciously, not mechanically. An attentive eye will perhaps notice a little difference but the greatest difference lies in the will they put into it, the consciousness they put into it. Walking to go somewhere and walking as an exercise is not the same thing. It is the conscious will in all these things which is important, it is that which brings about the progress and obtains the result. Therefore, what I mean is that the method one uses has only a relative importance in itself; it is the will to obtain a certain result that is important.

The yogi or aspiring yogi who does *asanas* to obtain a spiritual result or even simply a control over his body, obtains these results because it is with this aim that he does them, whereas I know some people who do exactly the same things but for all sorts of reasons unrelated to spiritual development, and who haven't even managed to acquire good health by it! And yet they do exactly the same thing, sometimes they even do it much better than the yogi, but it doesn't give them a stable health... because they haven't thought about it, haven't done it with this purpose in mind. I have asked them myself, I said, "But how can you be ill after doing all that?" — "Oh! but I never thought of it, that's not why I do it." This amounts to saying that it is the conscious will which acts on matter, not the material fact.

But you only have to try it, you will understand very well what I mean. For instance, all the movements you make when dressing, taking your bath, tidying your room... no matter what; make them consciously, with the will that this muscle should work, that muscle work. You will see, you will obtain really amazing results.

Going up and down the stairs — you cannot imagine how useful that can be from the point of view of physical culture, if you know how to make use of it. Instead of going up because you are going up and coming down because you are coming down, like any ordinary man, you go up with the consciousness of all the muscles which are working and of making them work harmoniously. You will see. Just try a little, you will see! This means that you can use all the movements of your life for a harmonious development of your body.

You bend down to pick something up, you stretch up to find something right at the top of a cupboard, you open a door, you close it, you have to go round an obstacle, there are a hundred and one things you do constantly and which you can make use of for your physical culture and which will demonstrate to you that it is the consciousness you put into it which produces the effect, a hundred times more than just the material fact of doing it. So, you choose the method you like best, but you can use the whole of your daily life in this way.... To think constantly of the harmony of the body, of the beauty of the movements, of not doing anything that is ungraceful and awkward. You can obtain a rhythm of movement and gesture which is very exceptional.

17 July 1957

An Enlightened Use of Human Will

It is good to utilise all that we have in order to increase and make more exact the control of physical activities. It is very obvious that those who practise physical culture scientifically and with coordination acquire a control over their bodies that's unimaginable for ordinary people. When the Russian gymnasts came here, we saw with what ease they did exercises which for an ordinary man are impossible, and they did them as if it was the simplest thing in the world; there was not even the least sign of effort! Well, that mastery is already a great step towards the transformation of the body. And these people who, I could say, are materialists by profession, used no spiritual method in their education; it was solely by material means and an enlightened use of human will that they had achieved this result. If they had added to this a spiritual knowledge and power, they could have achieved an almost miraculous result.... Because of the false ideas prevalent in the world, we don't usually see the two things together, spiritual mastery and material mastery, and so one is always incomplete without the other; but this is exactly what we want to do ... : if the two are combined, the result can reach a perfection that's unthinkable for the ordinary human mind, and this is what we want to attempt.

17 April 1957

Concentration and Dispersion

In sporting activities those who want to be successful choose a certain line or subject which appeals more to them and suits their nature; they concentrate on their choice and take great care not to disperse their energies in different directions. As in life a man chooses his career and concentrates all his attention upon it, so the sportsman chooses a special activity and concentrates all his efforts to achieve as much perfection as he can in this line. This perfection comes usually by a building up of spontaneous reflex which is the result of constant repetition of the same movements. But this spontaneous reflex can be, with advantage, replaced by the faculty of concentrated attention. This faculty of concentration belongs not only to the intellectual but to all activities and is obtained by the conscious control of the energies.

It is well known that the value of a man is in proportion to his capacity of concentrated attention, the greater the concentration the more exceptional is the result, to the extent that a perfect and unfailing concentrated attention sets the stamp of genius on what is produced. There can be genius in sports as in any other human activity.

Shall we then advise a limit to one action in order to achieve perfection in concentration?

The advantages of limitation are well known, but it has also its inconvenience, bringing narrowness and incapacity for any other line than the one chosen. This is contrary to the ideal of a perfectly developed and harmonised human being. How to conciliate these two contrary tendencies?

There seems to be only one solution to the problem. In the same way as an athlete develops methodically his muscles by a scientific and gradual training, the faculty of concentrated attention can be developed scientifically by a methodical training — developed in such a way that concentration is obtained at will and on whatever subject or activity is chosen. Thus the work of preparation instead of being done in the subconscient by a slow and steady repetition of the same movements, is done consciously by a concentration of will and a gathered attention centred on one point or another according to plan and decision. The chief difficulty seems to be to obtain this power of concentration independent from all inner and outer circumstances — difficult perhaps but not impossible for him who is determined and persevering. Moreover, whatever method of development is chosen, determination and perseverance are indispensable to obtain success.

The aim in the training is to develop this power of concentrating the attention at will on whatever subject or activity one chooses from the most spiritual to the most material, without losing anything of the fulness of the power, — for instance, in the physical field, transferring the use of the power from one game to another or one activity to another so as to succeed equally in all.

This extreme attention concentrated on a game or a physical activity like lifting, vaulting, punching, running, etc., focussing all energies on any of these movements which bring about in the body the thrill of an exhilarating joy is the thing which carries with it perfection in execution and success. Generally this happens when the sportsman is especially interested in a game or an activity and its happening escapes all control, decision or will.

Yet by a proper training of concentrated attention one can obtain the phenomenon at will, on command, so to say, and the resulting perfection in the execution of any activity follows inevitably.

This is exactly what we want to try in our Department of Physical Education. By this process the result may come more slowly than by the usual method, but the lack of rapidity will surely be compensated by a fulness and richness in the expression.

Bulletin, April 1949

Always Try a Little More

"The more you give, the more you receive," it is said. Does this apply to physical energy? Should one undertake physical work which seems beyond one's capacity? And what should be one's attitude while doing this kind of work?

If one did not spend, one would never receive. The great force a child has for growth, for development is that he spends without stint.

Naturally, when one spends, one must recuperate and must have the time that is needed to recuperate; but what a child cannot do one day, he can do the next. So if you never go beyond the limit you have reached, you will never progress. It is quite obvious that people who practise physical culture, for example, if they make progress, it is just because they gradually exceed, go beyond what they could do.

It is all a matter of balance. And the period of receptivity should be in proportion to the period of expenditure.

But if one confines oneself to what one can do at a given moment... First of all it is impossible, for if one doesn't progress, one falls back. Therefore, one must *always* make a little effort to do a little more than before. Then one is on the upward path. If one is afraid of doing too much, one is sure to go down again and lose one's capacities.

One must always try a little more, a little better than one did the day before or the previous moment. Only, the more one increases one's effort, the more should one increase one's capacity of receptivity and the opportunities to receive. For instance, from the purely physical point of view, if one wants to develop one's muscles, a progressive effort must be made by them, that is to say, a greater and greater effort, but at the same time one must do what is needed: massage, hydrotherapy, etc. to increase at the same time their capacity to receive.

And rest. A rest which is not a falling into the inconscient — which generally tires you more than it refreshes — but a conscious rest, a concentration in which one opens oneself and absorbs the forces which come, the universal forces.

The limits of the body's possibilities are so elastic! People who undergo a methodical and scientific training, rational, systematic, arrive at absolutely startling results. They demand things from their bodies which, naturally, without training it would be quite impossible to do. And certainly, they must gradually go beyond what they could do, not only from the point of view of perfection, but also from the point of view of strength. If they have that fear of doing more than they are able, of overdoing things, they will never progress. Only, at the same time one must do what is necessary for recuperating. That is the whole principle of physical culture. And one sees things which for an ignorant and untrained man are absolutely miraculous, performed by bodies which have been methodically trained.

20 June 1956

Is It Good to Force One's Body?

Mother, I have seen that I am not able to force my body to do a little better than my actual capacity. I would like to know how I can force it. But, Mother, is it good to force one's body?

No.

The body is capable of progressing and gradually it can learn to do what it could not do. But its capacity for progress is much slower than the vital desire for progress and the mind's will for progress. And if the vital and the mental were left masters of action, they would simply harass the body, destroy its poise and upset its health.

Therefore, one must be patient and follow the rhythm of one's body; it is more reasonable and knows what it can do and what it cannot.

Naturally, there are tamasic bodies and they need some encouragement for progressing.

But in everything and in all cases, one must keep one's balance.

13 October 1969

Physical Activities: An Offering to the Divine

Sweet Mother,
You have often told us that our activities must be an offering to the Divine. What does it mean exactly, and how to do it? For instance, when one plays tennis or basketball, how does one do that as an offering? Mental formations are not enough, naturally!

It means that what you do should not be done with a personal, egoistic aim, for success, for glory, for gain, for material profit or out of vanity, but as a service and an offering, in order to become more conscious of the divine will and to give oneself more entirely to it, until one has made enough progress to know and *feel* that it is the Divine who acts in you, His force that animates you and His will that supports you — not only a mental knowledge, but the sincerity of a state of consciousness and the power of a living experience.

For that to be possible, all egoistic motives and all egoistic reactions must disappear.

20 November 1961

Messages for Competitions

ATHLETICS COMPETITION 1962

Replace the ambition to be first by the will to do the best possible.

Replace the desire for success by the yearning for progress.

Replace the eagerness for fame by the aspiration for perfection.

Physical Education is meant to bring into the body consciousness and control, discipline and mastery, all things necessary for a higher and better life.

Keep all that in mind, practise sincerely and you will become a good athlete; this is the first step on the way to be a true man.

15 July 1962

ATHLETICS COMPETITION 1963

To all those who want to make their body fit for a Divine Life, I say, do not miss this excellent opportunity of the athletic competition and never forget that whatever we do we must aspire for perfection. For it is this yearning for perfection which will, in spite of all difficulties, lead us to our Goal.

Blessings.

21 August 1963

ATHLETICS COMPETITION 1964

We are here to lay the foundations of a new world.

All the virtues and skills required to succeed in athletics are exactly those the physical man must have to be fit for receiving and manifesting the new force.

I expect that with this knowledge and in this spirit you will enter this athletic competition and go through it successfully.

My blessings are with you.

24 August 1964

COMPETITIONS 1966

It might be better to remind you that we are here for a special work, a work which is done nowhere else.

We want to come in contact with the supreme consciousness, the universal consciousness, we want to bring it down in ourselves and to manifest it. But for that we must have a very solid base; our base is our physical being, our body. Therefore we have to build up a body solid, healthy, enduring, skilful, agile and strong, ready for everything. There is no better way to prepare the body than physical exercise: sports, athletics, gymnastics, and all games are the best means to develop and strengthen the body.

Therefore I call you to go through the competitions beginning to-day, fullheartedly with all your energy and all your will.

1 April 1966

COMPETITIONS 1967

On this occasion of our physical education and sportive activities:

I must tell you once more that for us spiritual life does not mean contempt for Matter but its divinisation. We do not want to reject the body but to transform it. For this physical education is one of the means most directly effective.

So I invite you to participate in the programme beginning today with enthusiasm and discipline — discipline, because it is the indispensable condition of order; enthusiasm, because it is the essential condition of success.

Blessings.

1 April 1967

COMPETITIONS 1968

The first condition for acquiring power is to be obedient.

The body must learn to obey before it can manifest power; and physical education is the most thorough discipline for the body.

So be eager and sincere in your efforts for physical education and you will acquire a powerful body.

My blessings are with you.

1 April 1968

COMPETITIONS 1969

Since the beginning of this year a new consciousness is at work upon earth to prepare the men for a new creation, the superman. For this creation to be possible the substance that constitutes man's body must undergo a big change, it must become more receptive to the consciousness and more plastic under its working.

These are just the qualities that one can acquire through physical education.

So, if we follow this discipline with such a result in view, we are sure to obtain the most interesting result.

My blessings to all, for progress and achievement.

1 April 1969

COMPETITIONS 1970

What better offering can we make to the Divine, than to offer the skill of our growing bodies?

Let us offer our efforts towards perfection, and physical education will take for us a new meaning and a greater value.

The world is preparing for a new creation, let us help through physical education, by making our bodies stronger, more receptive and more plastic, on the way to physical transformation.

1 April 1970

COMPETITIONS 1971

We are at one of these "Hours of God", when the old bases get shaken, and there is a great confusion; but it is a wonderful opportunity for those who want to leap forward, the possibility of progress is exceptional.

Will you not be of those who take advantage of it?

Let your body be prepared through physical education for this great change!

My blessings to all.

1 April 1971

The prayer of the cells
in the body.

Now that, by the effect
of the Grace, we are slowly
emerging out of inconscience
and waking to a conscious
life, an ardent prayer
rises in us for more light,
more consciousness,

" O Supreme Lord of the universe,
we implore Thee, give us the
strength and the beauty, the
harmonious perfection needed
to be Thy divine instruments
upon earth."

About Hatha Yoga

From our experience we have found that a particular system of exercises cannot be stamped as the only Yogic type of exercises and we cannot definitely say that participation in those exercises only will help to gain health because they are Yogic exercises.

Any rational system of exercises suited on one's need and capacity will help the participant to improve in health. Moreover, it is the attitude that is more important. Any well-planned and scientifically arranged programme of exercises practised with Yogic attitude will become Yogic exercises and the person practising them will draw full benefit from the point of view of physical health and moral and spiritual uplift.

Bulletin, April 1959

To Women about Their Body

(Answers to some questions)

1. For God's sake can't you forget that you are a girl or a boy and try to become a human being?
2. Each idea (or system of ideas) is true in its own time and place. But if it tries to be exclusive or to persist even when its time is over, then it ceases to be true.

THE MOTHER

While handling children in the Group for Physical Education we meet certain problems with girl students. Most of these are suggestions put upon them by their friends, older girls, parents and the doctor. Please throw your light on the following questions so that we may be better equipped in our knowledge to execute our responsibilities more efficiently.

1. What attitude should a girl take towards her monthly periods?

2. Should a girl participate in her normal programme of Physical Education during her periods?

3. Why are some girls completely run down during their periods and suffer from pains in the lower back and abdomen while others may have slight or no inconvenience at all?

4. How can a girl overcome her suffering and pains during periods?

5. Do you think there should be different types of exercises for boys and girls? Will a girl bring harm on her genital organs by practising the so-called manly sports?

6. Will a girl's appearance change and become muscular like a man and make her look ugly if she practises vigorous exercises?

7. Will the practice of vigorous types of exercises bring difficulties in child-birth if the girls want to marry and have children afterwards?

8. What should be the ideal of Physical Education for a girl from the point of view of her sex?

9. What roles should man and woman play in our new way of life? What shall be the relation between them?

10. What should be the ideal of a woman's physical beauty?

Before answering your questions I wish to tell you something which you know no doubt, but which you must never forget if you wish to learn how to lead a wise life.

It is true that we are, in our inner being, a spirit, a living soul that holds within it the Divine and aspires to become it, to manifest it perfectly; it is equally true, for the moment at least, that in our most material external being, in our body, we are still an animal, a mammalian, of a higher order no doubt, but made like animals and subject to the laws of animal Nature.

You have been taught surely that one peculiarity of the mammal is that the female conceives the child, carries it and builds it up within herself until the moment when the young one, fully formed, comes out of the body of its mother and lives independently.

In view of this function Nature has provided the woman with an additional quantity of blood which has to be used for the child in the making. But as the use of this additional blood is not a constant need, when there is no child in the making, the surplus blood has to be thrown out to avoid excess and congestion. This is the cause of the monthly periods. It is a simple natural phenomenon, a result of the way in which woman has been made and there is no need to attach to it more importance than to the other functions of the body. It is not a disease and cannot be the cause of any weakness or real discomfort. Therefore a normal woman, one who is not ridiculously sensitive, should merely take the necessary precautions of cleanliness, never think of it any more and lead her daily life as usual without any change in her programme. This is the best way to be in good health.

Besides, even while recognising that in our body we still belong dreadfully to animality, we must not therefore conclude that this animal part, as it is the most concrete and the most real for us, is one to which we are obliged to be subjected and which we must allow to rule over us. Unfortunately this is what happens most often in life and men are certainly much more slaves than masters of their physical being. Yet it is the contrary that should be, for the truth of individual life is quite another thing.

We have in us an intelligent will more or less enlightened which is the first instrument of our psychic being. It is this intelligent will that we must use in order to learn to live not like an animal man, but as a human being, candidate for Divinity.

And the first step towards this realisation is to become master of this body instead of remaining an impotent slave.

One most effective help towards this goal is physical culture.

For about a century there has been a renewal of a knowledge greatly favoured in ancient times, partially forgotten since then. Now it is reawakening, and with the progress of modern science, it is acquiring quite a new amplitude and importance. This knowledge deals with the physical body and the extraordinary mastery that can be obtained over it with the help of enlightened and systematised physical education.

This renewal has been the result of the action of a new power and light that have spread upon the earth in order to prepare it for the great transformations that must take place in the near future.

We must not hesitate to give a primary importance to this physical education whose very purpose is to make our body capable of receiving and expressing the new force which seeks to manifest upon earth.

This said I now answer the questions you put to me.

1. What attitude should a girl take towards her monthly periods?

The attitude you take towards something quite natural and unavoidable. Give it as little importance as possible and go on with your usual life, without changing anything because of it.

2. Should a girl participate in her normal programme of Physical Education during her periods?

Certainly if she is accustomed to physical exercise, she must not stop because of that. If one keeps the habit of leading one's normal life always, very soon one does not even notice the presence of the menses.

3. Why are some girls completely run down during their periods and suffer from pain in the lower back and abdomen while others may have slight or no inconvenience at all?

It is a question of temperament and mostly of education. If from her childhood a girl has been accustomed to pay much attention to the slightest uneasiness and to make a big fuss about the smallest inconvenience, then she loses all capacity of endurance and anything becomes the occasion for being pulled down. Especially if the parents themselves get too easily anxious about the reactions of their children. It is wiser to teach a child to be a bit sturdy and enduring than to show much care for these small inconveniences and accidents that cannot always be avoided in life. An attitude of quiet forbearance is the best one can adopt for oneself and teach to the children.

It is a well-known fact that if you expect some pain you are bound to have it and, once it has come, if you concentrate upon it, then it increases more and more until it becomes what is usually termed as "unbearable", although with some will and courage there is hardly any pain that one cannot bear.

4. How can a girl overcome her suffering and pain during periods?

There are some exercises that make the abdomen strong and improve the circulation. These exercises must be done regularly and continued even after the pains have disappeared. For the grown up girls, this kind of pain comes almost entirely from sexual desires. If we get rid of the desires we get rid of the pains. There are two ways of getting rid of desires; the first one, the usual one, is through satisfaction (or rather what is called so, because there is no such thing as satisfaction in the domain of desire). That means leading the ordinary human-animal life, marriage, children and all the rest of it.

There is, of course, another way, a better way, — control, mastery, transformation; this is more dignified and also more effective.

5. Do you think there should be different types of exercises for boys and girls? Will a girl bring harm on her genital organs by practising the so-called manly sports?

In all cases, as well for boys as for girls, the exercises must be graded according to the strength and the capacity of each one. If a weak student tries at once to do hard and heavy exercises, he may suffer for his foolishness. But with a wise and progressive training, girls as well as boys can participate in all kinds of sports, and thus increase their strength and health.

To become strong and healthy can never bring harm to a body even if it is a woman's body.

6. Will a girl's appearance change and become muscular like a muscular man and make her look ugly if she practises vigorous exercises?

Weakness and fragility may look attractive in the view of a perverted mind, but it is not the truth of Nature nor the truth of the Spirit.

If you have ever looked at the photos of the women gymnasts you will know what perfectly beautiful bodies they have; and nobody can deny that they are muscular!

7. Will the practice of vigorous types of exercises bring difficulties in child-birth if the girls want to marry and have children afterwards?

I never came across such a case. On the contrary, women who are trained to strong exercises and have a muscular body go through the ordeal of child-formation and child-birth much more easily and painlessly.

I heard the authentic story of one of these African women who are accustomed to walk for miles carrying heavy loads. She was pregnant and the time of delivery came during one of the day's marches. She sat on the side of the track, under a tree, gave birth to the child, waited for half an hour, then she rose and adding the new born babe to the former luggage, went on her way quietly, as if nothing had happened. This is a splendid example of what a woman can do when she is in full possession of her health and strength.

Doctors will say that such a thing cannot occur in a civilised world with all the so-called progress that humanity has achieved; but we cannot deny that, from the physical point of view, this is a more happy condition than all the sensitiveness, the sufferings and the complications created by the modern civilisations.

Moreover, usually doctors are more interested in the abnormal cases, and they judge mostly from that point of view. But for us, it is different; it is from the normal that we can rise to the supernormal, not from the abnormal which is always a sign of perversion and inferiority.

8. What should be the ideal of Physical Education for a girl from the point of view of her sex?

I do not see why there should be any special ideal of physical education for girls other than for boys.

Physical education has for its aim to develop all the possibilities of a human body, possibilities of harmony, strength, plasticity, cleverness, agility, endurance, and to increase the control over the functioning of the limbs and the organs, to make of the body a perfect instrument at the disposal of a conscious will. This programme is excellent for all human beings equally, and there is no point in wanting to adopt another one for girls.

9. What roles should man and woman play in our new way of life? What shall be the relation between them?

Why make at all a distinction between them? They are all equally human beings, trying to become fit instruments for the Divine Work, above sex, caste, creed and nationality, all children of the same Infinite Mother and aspirants to the one Eternal Godhead.

10. What should be the ideal of a woman's physical beauty?

A perfect harmony in the proportions, suppleness and strength, grace and force, plasticity and endurance, and above all, an excellent health, unvarying and unchanging, which is the re-

sult of a pure soul, a happy trust in life and an unshakable faith
in the Divine Grace.

One word to finish:

I have told you these things, because you needed to hear
them, but do not make of them absolute dogmas, for that would
take away their truth.

1960

6

DIFFICULTIES

To Overcome Bodily Fear

*One is often afraid of doing what is new; the body refuses
to act in a new way, like trying a new gymnastic figure or
another way of diving. From where does this fear come?
How can one free oneself of it? And again, how can one
encourage others to do the same?*

The body is afraid of anything new because its very base is inertia, *tamas*; it is the vital which brings the dominance of *rajas*
(activity). That is why, generally, the intrusion of the vital in
the form of ambition, emulation and egotism, obliges the body
to shake off tamas and make the necessary effort to progress.

Naturally, those in whom the mind predominates can lec-
ture their body and provide it with all the necessary reasons
to enable it to overcome its fear.

The best way for everybody is self-giving to the Divine and
confidence in His infinite Grace.

Fear and Laziness

*If in gymnastics I want to take a jump and I feel fright-
ened, why does this happen?*

Ah! there, my children, it depends.... You must distinguish
two very different things and you must deal with them very
differently.

If it is a vital fear, you must reason with yourself and go about it all the same. But if it is a physical instinct (that is possible, it happens very often that there is a kind of physical instinct), in that case you must listen to it, for the instinct of the body is a very sure thing, if it is not disturbed by thought or vital will. The body left to itself knows very well what it can and what it cannot do. And not only that but even a thing that one can do and does usually, if one day you feel a sort of repulsion, as if you were shrinking back, you must definitely not do it; it is an indication that for some reason or other — a purely material reason of a disorder in the functioning of the body — you are not fit to do the thing at that time. Then you must not do it. In that case, it is not even a fear, it is something that shrinks, that withdraws, there is nothing in the head, it does not correspond to any kind of thought like: "What is going to happen?" When the head starts working and you say: "What is going to happen?", you must sweep it away because it is worth nothing; you must use all the means of reason and good sense you have to drive that away. But if it is a purely physical sensation, as though something were contracting, a kind of physical repugnance, if the body itself is refusing, so to say, you should never force it, never, because it is usually when you force it that there's an accident. That may very well be a kind of premonition that there's going to be an accident, that if you do the thing, you will not go far. And in such a case you must not do it. You must not put into it the least *amour-propre*. You must realise: "Today I am not in a good condition."

But if it is a vital fear, if for example you have a competition or a tournament, and you felt this kind of fear and then: "What is going to happen?", you must sweep it away quickly, it means nothing.

*But sometimes, it is laziness that prevents us from doing
a thing.*

Ah! if you are tamasic, that is yet something else. If you have
a tamasic nature, you must use another procedure. You must
exert your consciousness, your will, your force, gather your
energy, shake yourself a little and whip yourself and say:
"Clac! clac! forward, march." If it is laziness that keeps you
back from, say, doing the vaulting, you must immediately do
something much more tiring and say: "Well, you don't want to
do that? All right, you are going to do 1500 metres running!"
Or else: "I don't want to do the weight-lifting today, I don't
feel like doing it: good, I shall do skipping 4000 times at a
stretch." . . .

*Would it not be better to continue the work even if one feels
lazy?*

That depends on the work; there we enter another domain.
   If it is a work that you are doing for the collectivity and not
for yourself personally, then you must do it, whatever happens.
It is an elementary discipline. You have undertaken to do this
work or have been given the work and have taken it up, therefore you have accepted it, and in that case you must do it. At
all times, unless you are absolutely ill, ill in the last degree and
unable to move, you must do it. Even if you are rather ill, you
must do it. An unselfish work always cures you of your petty
personal maladies. Naturally, if you are really compelled to
be in bed without being able to move, with a terrible fever or
a very serious illness, then that's quite different. But otherwise, if you are just a little indisposed: "I am not feeling quite
well, I have a little headache or I have indigestion, or I have a
bad cold, I am coughing", things like that — then doing your

work, not thinking of yourself, thinking of the work, doing it
as well as you can, that puts you right immediately.

24 June 1953

Why Does the Body Get Tired?

*Why does the body get tired? We have more or less reg-
ular activities, but one day we are full of energy and the
next day we are quite tired.*

Generally this comes from a kind of inner disequilibrium.
There may be many reasons for it, but it all comes to this: a
sort of disequilibrium between the different parts of the being.
Now, it is also possible that the day one had the energy, one
spent it too much, though this is not the case with children;
children spend it until they can no longer do so. One sees a
child active till the moment he suddenly falls fast asleep. He
was there, moving, running; and then, all of a sudden, pluff!
finished, he is asleep. And it is in this way that he grows up,
becomes stronger and stronger. Consequently, it is not the
spending that harms you. The expenditure is made up by the
necessary rest — that is set right very well. No, it is a disequilibrium: the harmony between the different parts of the being
is no longer sufficient.

People think they have only to continue doing for ever what
they were doing or at least remain in the same state of consciousness, day after day do their little work, and all will go
well. But it is not like that. Suddenly, for some reason or
other, one part of the being — either your feelings or your
thoughts or your vital — makes progress, has discovered something, received a light, progressed. It takes a leap in progress.
All the rest remains behind. This brings about a disequili-

brium. That is enough to make you very tired. But in fact, it is not tiredness: it is something which makes you want to keep quiet, to concentrate, remain within yourself, be like that, and build up slowly a new harmony among the different parts of the being. And it is very necessary to have, at a given moment, a sort of rest, for an assimilation of what one has learnt and a harmonisation of the different parts of the being.

24 February 1954

Depression Cuts Every Source of Energy

When we play badly we find that we have no energy, but if we play well, with great enthusiasm, we find that energy comes. Why ?

This is perfectly true. To enter into contact with terrestrial energy, one must establish a certain harmony within oneself. If you know the game well, if you know how to make the moves and if you take an enthusiastic interest, if you have a sort of ambition (quite childish perhaps), a desire to win, then as you go on succeeding you feel a kind of inner joy, not perhaps very profound, but creating the harmony necessary for the interchange of energy. On the other hand, those who do not know how to accept defeat, who get angry and bad-tempered when things do not go according to their wish, lose their energy more and more.

Also, if you slip into depression, you cut every source of energy — from above, from below, from everywhere. That is the best way of falling into inertia. You must absolutely refuse to be depressed.

Depression is always the sign of an acute egoism. When

you feel that it is coming near, tell yourself: "I am in a state of egoistic illness, I must cure myself of it."

25 December 1950

How Can Depression Be Controlled?

How can depressions be controlled?

Oh! there's a very simple way. Depression occurs generally in the vital, and one is overpowered by depression only when one keeps the consciousness in the vital, when one remains there. The only thing to do is to get out of the vital and enter a deeper consciousness. Even the higher mind, the luminous, higher mind, the most lofty thoughts have the power to drive away depression. Even when one reaches just the highest domains of thought, usually the depression disappears. But in any case, if one seeks shelter in the psychic, then there is no longer any room for depression.

Depression may come from two causes: either from a want of vital satisfaction or from a considerable nervous fatigue in the body. Depression arising from physical fatigue is set right fairly easily: one has but to take rest. One goes to bed and sleeps until one feels well again, or else one rests, dreams, lies down. The want of vital satisfaction is pretty easily produced and usually one must face it with one's reason, must ferret out the cause of the depression, what has brought about the lack of satisfaction in the vital; and then one looks at it straight in the face and asks oneself whether that indeed has anything to do with one's inner aspiration or whether it is simply quite an ordinary movement. Generally one discovers that it has nothing to do with the inner aspiration and one can quite easily overcome it and resume one's normal movement. If that does not suffice, then one must go deeper and deeper until one touches the psychic reality. Then one has only to put this psychic reality in contact with the movement of depression, and instantaneously it will vanish into thin air.

24 February 1954

Mastery of Depression

Is it the same thing, the same work, to be conscious that the nature must be changed and to master the different parts of the being?

One precedes the other. First of all one must be conscious, then control, and by continuing the mastery one changes one's character. Changing the character is what comes last. One must control bad habits, the old habits, for a very long time for them to drop off and the character to change.

We may take the example of someone who has frequent depressions. When things are not exactly as he would like them to be, he becomes depressed. So, to begin with, he must become aware of his depression — not only of the depression but of the causes of depression, why he gets depressed so easily. Then, once he has become conscious, he must master the depressions, must stop being depressed even when the cause of depression is there — he must master his depression, stop it from coming. And finally, after this work has been done for a sufficiently long time, the nature loses the habit of having depressions and no longer reacts in the same way, the nature is changed.

21 April 1951

Waste of Energy

Human beings do not know how to preserve energy. When something happens, an accident or an illness, help is asked for and a double or triple dose of energy is administered. They feel themselves to be receptive and they receive it. This energy is given for two reasons: to repair the disorder caused by the accident or illness and to give the strength for transformation, to mend, to change what was the true cause of the illness or accident.

Instead of utilising energy in that way, immediately, forthwith they throw it outside. They begin to move about, to be active, to work. They begin to speak, they begin to say... they feel themselves full of energy and throw everything outside! They can keep nothing. Then naturally, as the energy was not meant to be wasted like that, but for an inner use, they fall quite flat. And this is universal. They do not know, they do not know how to make that movement: to go within, utilise the energy — not to keep it, it cannot be kept — utilise it to mend the damage done to the body and to go deep down to find out the reason for the accident or the malady, and there to change that into an aspiration, an inner transformation. Instead of this, people begin immediately to prattle, to move about, to work, to do this, to do that!

Indeed, the great majority of human beings feel that they are alive only when they waste energy, otherwise it does not look like life.

Not to waste energy means to utilise it for the purposes for which it was given. If the energy is given for transformation, for the sublimation of the being, it must be used for that; if the energy is given to set right something that has been disorganised in the body, it must be used for that.

Naturally, if someone is given a special work and if he is

given the energy to do that work, it is all right, it is used for its purposes; but it was given for that.

As soon as man feels energetic, he rushes forthwith into action. Or otherwise, those who have not got the sense of any useful thing, they gossip. Worse still, they who have no control upon themselves become intolerant and begin to dispute! If their will is contradicted, they feel themselves full of energy and take that as holy wrath!

The "Need" of Relaxation

Everything comes from this "need" of relaxation; and what does that mean for most men? It means, always, coming down to a lower level. They do not know that for a true relaxation one must rise one degree higher, one must rise above oneself. If one goes down, it adds to one's fatigue and brings a stupefaction. Besides, each time one comes down, one increases the load of the subconscient — this huge subconscient load which one must clean and clean if one wants to mount, and which is like fetters on the feet. But it is difficult to teach that, for one must know it oneself before one can teach it to others.

This is never told to children, they are allowed to commit all the stupidities in the world under the pretext that they need relaxation.

It is not by sinking below oneself that one removes fatigue. One must climb the ladder and there one has true rest, because one has the inner peace, the light, the universal energy. And little by little one puts oneself in touch with the truth which is the very reason of one's existence.

If you contact that definitively, it removes completely all fatigue.

26 February 1951

Boredom: The Most Common Human Malady

To tell the truth, the most common malady humanity suffers from is boredom. Most of the stupidities men commit come from an attempt to escape boredom. Well, I say for certain that no outer means are any good, and that boredom pursues you and will pursue you no matter what you try in order to escape from it, but this way, that is, beginning this work of organising your being and all its movements and all its elements around the central Consciousness and Presence, this is the surest and most complete cure, and the most comforting, for all possible boredom. It gives a tremendous interest. And an extraordinary diversity. You no longer have the time to get bored.

6 June 1956

Fatigue Comes from Doing without Interest

Fatigue comes from doing without interest the things you do.

Whatever you do you can find interest in it, provided you take it as the means of progressing; you must try to do better and better what you are doing, the will for progress must always be there and then you take interest in what you do, whatever it is. The most insignificant occupation can prove interesting if you take it that way.

But even the most attractive and important activity will soon lose all its interest for you if the will for progress towards an ideal perfection is not there while you act.

*

Tiredness shows lack of will for progress. When you feel tired or fatigued that is lack of will for progress.

7

SOURCES OF ENERGY

Effort Gives Joy

An aim gives a meaning, a purpose to life, and this purpose implies an effort; and it is in effort that one finds joy.

Exactly. It is the effort which gives joy; a human being who does not know how to make an effort will never find joy. Those who are essentially lazy will never find joy — they do not have the strength to be joyful! It is effort which gives joy. Effort makes the being vibrate at a certain degree of tension which makes it possible for you to feel the joy. . . .

It is only effort, in whatever domain it be — material effort, moral effort, intellectual effort — which creates in the being certain vibrations which enable you to get connected with universal vibrations; and it is this which gives joy. It is effort which pulls you out of inertia; it is effort which makes you receptive to the universal forces. And the one thing above all which spontaneously gives joy, even to those who do not practise yoga, who have no spiritual aspiration, who lead quite an ordinary life, is the exchange of forces with universal forces. People do not know this, they would not be able to tell you that it is due to this, but so it is.

13 January 1951

Energy Inexhaustible

One of the most powerful aids that yogic discipline can provide to the sportsman is to teach him how to renew his energies by drawing them from the inexhaustible source of universal energy.

Modern science has made great progress in the art of nourishment, which is the best known means of replenishing one's energies. But this process is at best precarious and subject to all kinds of limitations. We shall not speak about it here, for the subject has already been discussed at great length. But it is quite obvious that so long as the world and men are what they are, food is an indispensable factor. Yogic science knows of other ways of acquiring energy, and we shall mention two of the most important.

The first is to put oneself in relation with the energies accumulated in the terrestrial material world and to draw freely from this inexhaustible source. These material energies are obscure and half unconscious; they encourage animality in man, but, at the same time, they establish a kind of harmonious relationship between the human being and material Nature. Those who know how to receive and use these energies are usually successful in life and succeed in everything they undertake. But they are still largely dependent on their living conditions and their state of bodily health. The harmony created in them is not immune from all attack; it usually vanishes when circumstances become adverse. The child spontaneously receives this energy from material Nature as he expends all his energies without calculating, joyfully and freely. But in most human beings, as they grow up, this faculty is blunted by the worries of life, as a result of the predominant place which mental activities come to occupy in the consciousness.

However, there is a source of energy which, once discovered, is never exhausted, whatever the outer circumstances and physical conditions of life may be. It is the energy that can be described as spiritual, which is received no longer from below, from the inconscient depths, but from above, from the supreme origin of the universe and man, from the all-powerful and eternal splendours of the superconscient. It is there, all around us, permeating everything; and to enter into contact with it and to receive it, it is enough to aspire sincerely for it, to open oneself to it in faith and trust, to widen one's consciousness and identify it with the universal Consciousness.

At the outset, this may seem very difficult, if not impossible. Yet by examining this phenomenon more closely, one can see that it is not so alien, not so remote from the normally developed human consciousness. Indeed, there are very few people who have not felt, at least once in their lives, as if lifted up beyond themselves, filled with an unexpected and uncommon force which, for a time, has made them capable of doing anything whatever; at such moments nothing seems too difficult and the word "impossible" loses its meaning.

This experience, however fleeting it may be, gives a glimpse of the kind of contact with the higher energy that yogic discipline can secure and maintain.

The method of achieving this contact can hardly be given here. Besides, it is something individual and unique for each one, which starts from where he stands, adapting itself to his personal needs and helping him to take one more step forward. The path is sometimes long and slow, but the result is worth the trouble one takes. We can easily imagine the consequences of this power to draw at will and in all circumstances on the boundless source of an energy that is all-powerful in its luminous purity. Weariness, exhaustion, illness, old age and even death become mere obstacles on the way, which a persistent will is sure to overcome.

Bulletin, August 1949

Three Sources of Subsistence

"The vital has three sources of subsistence. The one most easily accessible to it comes from below, from the physical energies through the sensations.

"The second is on its own plane, when it is sufficiently vast and receptive, by contact with the universal vital forces.

"The third, to which it usually opens only in a great aspiration for progress, comes to it from above by the infusion and absorption of spiritual forces and inspiration. . . ."

The Mother, "The Four Austerities"

There are three sources, you know. The third source is usually closed to people; it comes to them only in moments of great aspiration. When they have a very great aspiration and rise towards higher forces, at that time the vital can receive these higher forces into itself; and then this becomes a source of considerable energy for it. But in its ordinary, habitual life it is not in contact with these forces — unless, of course, it is transformed; but I am speaking of the ordinary vital in ordinary life. It is not open to this source of higher forces, and for it this is even altogether non-existent. In the immense majority of people all their vital force comes to them from below, from the earth, from food, from all the sensations. From food... they draw vital energy out of food, and they... it is by seeing, hearing, touching, feeling that they contact the energies contained in matter. They draw them in this way. This is their customary food.

Now, some people have a very developed vital which they have subjected to a discipline — and they have a sense of immensity and are in contact with the world and the movements of world-forces. And so they can receive... if in a movement of calling... they can receive the universal vital forces which enter them and renew the dose of energy they need.

There are others, very rare ones — or may be in very rare moments of their individual life — who have an aspiration for the higher consciousness, higher force, higher knowledge, and who, by this call, draw to themselves the forces of higher domains. And so this also renews in them very special energies, of a special value.

But unless one is practising yoga, a regular discipline, usually one does not often contact this source; one draws from the same level or from below.

31 March 1954

The Capacity to Cure Oneself

Mother, is it possible to develop in oneself the capacity to cure oneself?

All is possible in principle by uniting oneself consciously with the Divine Force.

But a procedure has to be found and that depends upon cases and individuals.

The first condition is to have a physical nature that pours out energy instead of drawing energy from others.

The second indispensable condition is to know how to

draw energy from above, from the impersonal inexhaustible source.

In this way the more one spends the more one receives and one becomes an inexhaustible channel and not a vessel that empties itself by giving.

It is through a steadfast aspiration that one learns.

12 and 13 January 1972

PART IV

THE CYCLE OF LIFE

I

BIRTH

The Mother and Father Can Call a Soul

Sweet Mother, is it possible for the mother and father to give birth to... to ask for the soul they want?

To ask? For that they must have an occult knowledge which they don't usually have. But anyway, what is possible is that instead of doing the thing like an animal driven by instinct or desire and most of the time, without even wanting it, they do it at will, with an aspiration, putting themselves in a state of aspiration and almost of prayer, so that the being they are going to form may be one fit to embody a soul which they *can* call down to incarnate in that form. I knew people — not many, this does not often happen, but still I knew some — who chose special circumstances, prepared themselves through special concentration and meditation and aspiration and sought to bring down, into the body they were going to form, an exceptional being.

In many countries of old — and even now in certain countries — the woman who was going to have a child was placed in special conditions of beauty, harmony, peace and well-being, in very harmonious physical conditions, so that the child could be formed in the best possible conditions. This is obviously what ought to be done, for it is within the reach of human possibilities. Human beings are developed enough for this not to be something quite exceptional. And yet it is quite exceptional, for very few people think of it, while there are *innumerable* people who have children without even wanting to.

That was what I wanted to say.

It is possible to call a soul, but one must be at least a little conscious oneself, and must want to do what one does in the best conditions. This is very rare, but it is possible.

27 June 1956

Willed Conception Is Extremely Rare

I have said what kind of aspiration ought to be there in the parents before the birth; but as I said, this does not happen even once in a hundred thousand instances. The willed conception of a child is extremely rare; mostly it is an accident. Among innumerable parents it is quite a small minority that even simply bothers about what a child could be; they do not even know that what the child will be depends on what they are. It is a very small *élite* which knows this. Most of the time things go as they can; anything at all happens and people don't even realise what is happening.

29 March 1951

True Maternity

Maternity is considered as the principal role of woman. But this is true only so long as we understand what is meant by the word maternity. For to bring children into the world as rabbits do their young — instinctively, ignorantly, machine-like, that certainly cannot be called maternity! True maternity begins with the conscious creation of a being, with the willed shaping of a soul coming to develop and utilise a new body. The true domain of women is the spiritual. We forget it but too often.

To bear a child and construct his body almost subconsciously is not enough. The work really commences when, by the power of thought and will, we conceive and create a character capable of manifesting an ideal.

And do not say that we have no power for realising such a thing. Innumerable instances of this very effective power could be brought out as proofs.

First of all, the effect of physical environment was recognised and studied long ago. It is by surrounding women with forms of art and beauty that, little by little, the ancient Greeks created the exceptionally harmonious race that they were.

Individual instances of the same fact are numerous. It is not rare to see a woman who, while pregnant, had looked at constantly and admired a beautiful picture or statue, giving birth to a child after the perfect likeness of this picture or statue. I met several of these instances myself. Among them, I remember very clearly two little girls; they were twins and perfectly beautiful. But the most astonishing was how little like their parents they were. They reminded me of a very famous picture painted by the English artist Reynolds. One day I made this remark to the mother, who immediately exclaimed: "Indeed, is it not so? You will be interested to know that while I was expecting these children, I had, hanging above my bed, a very good reproduction of Reynold's picture. Before going to sleep and as soon I woke, my last and first glance was for that picture; and in my heart I hoped: may my children be like the faces in this picture. You see that I succeeded quite well!" In truth, she could be proud of her success, and her example is of great utility for other women.

But if we can obtain such results on the physical plane where the materials are the least plastic, how much more so on the psychological plane where the influence of thought and will is so powerful. Why accept the obscure bonds of heredity and atavism — which are nothing else than subconscious preferences for our own trend of character — when we can, by concentration and will, call into being a type constructed according to the highest ideal we are able to conceive? With this effort, maternity becomes truly precious and sacred; indeed with this, we enter the glorious work of the Spirit, and womanhood rises above animality and its ordinary instincts, towards real humanity and its powers.

A Mother's Aspiration and Will

The education of a human being should begin at birth and continue throughout his life.

Indeed, if we want this education to have its maximum result, it should begin even before birth; in this case it is the mother herself who proceeds with this education by means of a twofold action: first, upon herself for her own improvement, and secondly, upon the child whom she is forming physically. For it is certain that the nature of the child to be born depends very much upon the mother who forms it, upon her aspiration and will as well as upon the material surroundings in which she lives. To see that her thoughts are always beautiful and pure, her feelings always noble and fine, her material surroundings as harmonious as possible and full of a great simplicity — this is the part of education which should apply to the mother herself. And if she has in addition a conscious and definite will to form the child according to the highest ideal she can conceive, then the very best conditions will be realised so that the child can come into the world with his utmost potentialities. How many difficult efforts and useless complications would be avoided in this way!

February 1951

The Incarnation of Evolved Souls

I may say that I have been present at innumerable incarnations of evolved souls in beings either preparing to be born or already born. As I said, the cases are quite different; it depends more on psychological conditions than on material ones, but it also depends on material conditions. It depends on the state of development of the soul which wants to reincarnate — we take the word "soul" here in the sense of the psychic being, what we call the psychic being — it depends on its state of development, on the milieu in which it is going to incarnate, on the mission it has to fulfil — that makes many different conditions…. It depends very largely on the state of consciousness of the parents. For it goes without saying that there is a stupendous difference between conceiving a child deliberately, with a conscious aspiration, a call to the invisible world and a spiritual ardour, and conceiving a child by accident and without intending to have it, and sometimes even without wanting it at all. I don't say that in the latter case there cannot also be an incarnation, but it usually takes place later, not at the conception.

For the formation of the child it makes a great difference.

If the incarnation takes place at the conception, the whole formation of the child to be born is directed and governed by the consciousness which is going to incarnate: the choice of the elements, the attraction of the substance — a choice of the forces and even the substance of the matter which is assimilated. There is already a selection. And this naturally creates altogether special conditions for the formation of the body, which may already be fairly developed, evolved, harmonised before its birth. I must say that this is quite, quite exceptional; but still it does happen.

More frequently there are cases in which, just at the moment of its birth, that is to say, of its first gesture of independence, when the child begins to develop its lungs by crying as much as it can, at that moment, very often, this sort of call from life makes the descent easier and more effective.

Sometimes days and at times months pass, and the preparation is slow and the entry takes place very gradually, in quite a subtle and almost imperceptible way.

Sometimes it comes much later, when the child itself becomes a little conscious and feels a very subtle but very real relation with something from above, far above, which is like an influence pressing upon it; and then it can begin to feel the need of being in contact with this something which it does not know, does not understand, but which it can only feel; and this aspiration draws the psychic and makes it descend into the child.

I am giving you here a few fairly common instances; there are many others; this may happen in innumerable different ways. What I have described to you are the most frequent cases I have seen.

So, the soul which wants to incarnate stays at times in a domain of the higher mind, quite close to the earth, having chosen its future home; or else it can descend further, into the vital, and from there have a more direct action; or again it can enter the subtle physical and very closely govern the development of its future body.

24 October 1956

Do Great Souls Choose Their Parents ?

When great souls want to be born upon earth, do they choose their parents ?

Ah! that depends on their state of consciousness, it depends on the state of their psychic formation. If the psychic being is completely formed, if it has reached the perfection of its being and is free to reincarnate or not, it has also the capacity of choosing. But I believe I have explained that to you already. They don't have a physical sight like ours so long as they are not in a body. So, evidently, they look for a body which is adapted and fit to express them, but they must give its share to the material inconscience, if it may be put thus, and to the necessity to adapt themselves to the most material laws of the body. So, from the point of view of the psychic, the choice of the place where one is born is important, it is more than an insignificant detail. But there are so many things that can't be foreseen. For instance, one chooses an environment, a country, a certain type of family, one tries to see the nature of the probable parents, one asks for certain already well-developed qualities in them and a sufficient self-mastery. But all this is not enough if one does not carry in oneself a sufficient dynamism to overcome the obstacles. So, all things considered, this is not enormously important. Anyhow, even at the best, even if the parents have collaborated consciously, there is an enormous mass of the subconscient and the yet lower inconscient which from time to time rises again to the surface, gets stirred up, damages the work, makes calmness and silence indispensable. Always, always a preparation is needed, even if one has chosen — a long preparation. Not to speak of the phenomenon of being half-stunned at the moment of birth, the descent into the body, which often lasts for a very long time before one can escape from it completely.

30 December 1953

The Developed Psychic Being Chooses Its Conditions

There comes a moment when this psychic being is sufficiently developed to have an independent consciousness and a personal will. And then after innumerable lives more or less individualised, it becomes conscious of itself, of its movements and of the environment it has chosen for its growth. Arriving at a certain state of perception, it decides — generally at the last minute of the life it has just finished upon earth — the conditions in which its next life will be passed. . . . After having finished one life (which usually ends only when it has done what it wanted to do), it will have chosen the environment where it will be born, the approximate place where it will be born, the conditions and the kind of life in which it will be born, and a very precise programme of the experiences through which it will have to pass to be able to make the progress it wants to make.

I am going to give you quite a concrete example. Let us take a psychic being that has decided, for some reason or other, to enter the body of a being destined to become king, because there is a whole series of experiences it can have only under those conditions. After having passed through these experiences of a king, it finds that there is a whole domain in which it cannot make a progress due to these very conditions of life where it is. So when it has finished its term upon earth and decides to go away, it decides that in its next life it will take birth in an ordinary environment and in ordinary conditions, neither high nor low, but such that the body which it will take up will be free to do what it likes. For I do not tell you anything new when I say that the life of a king is the life of a slave; a king is obliged to submit to a whole protocol and to all kinds of ceremonies to keep his prestige (it is perhaps very pleasant for vain people, but for a psychic being it is not pleasant, for

this deprives it of the possibility of a large number of experiences). So having taken this decision, it carries in itself all
the memories which a royal life can give it and it takes rest for
the period it considers necessary (here, I must say that I am
speaking of a psychic being exclusively occupied with itself,
not one consecrated to a work, because in that case it is
the work which decides the future lives and their conditions; I am speaking of a psychic being at work completing
its development). Hence it decides that at a certain moment
it will take a body. Having already had a number of experiences, it knows that in a certain country, a certain part of the
consciousness has developed; in another, another part, and
so on; so it chooses the place which offers it easy possibilities
of development: the country, the conditions of living, the approximate nature of the parents, and also the condition of the
body itself, its physical structure and the qualities it needs for
its experiences. It takes rest, then at the required moment
wakes up and projects its consciousness upon earth centralis-
ing it in the chosen domain and the chosen conditions — or
almost so; there is a small margin you know, for in the psychic
consciousness one is too far away from the material physical
consciousness to be able to see with a clear vision; it is an ap-
proximation. It does not make a mistake about the country or
the environment and it sees quite clearly the inner vibrations
of the people chosen, but there may happen to be a slight in-
decision. But if, just at this moment, there is a couple upon
earth or rather a woman who has a psychic aspiration herself
and, for some reason or other, without knowing why or how,
would like to have an exceptional child, answering certain exceptional conditions; if at this moment there is this aspiration
upon earth, it creates a vibration, a psychic light which the
psychic being sees immediately and, without hesitation it
rushes towards it. Then, from that moment (which is the mo-

ment of conception), it watches over the formation of the child, so that this formation may be as favourable as possible to the plan it has; consequently its influence is there over the child even before it appears in the physical world.

If all goes well, if there is no accident (accidents can always happen), if all goes well at the moment the child is about to be born, the psychic force (perhaps not in its totality, but a part of the psychic consciousness) rushes into the being and from its very first cry gives it a push towards the experiences it wants the child to acquire. The result is that even if the parents are not conscious, even if the child in its external consciousness is not quite conscious (a little child does not have the necessary brain for that, it forms slowly, little by little), in spite of that, it will be possible for the psychic influence to direct all the events, all the circumstances of the life of this child till the moment it becomes capable of coming into conscious contact with its psychic being (physically it is generally between the age of four and seven, sometimes sooner, sometimes almost immediately, but in such a case we deal with children who are not "children", who have "supernatural" qualities, as they say — they are not "supernatural", but simply the expression of the presence of the psychic being).

24 February 1951

A Precise Place to Take Birth

Can it happen that the psychic being does not fall at the place where it wanted to take birth?

If a psychic being sees from its psychic world a light on the earth, it may rush down there without knowing exactly where it is. Everything is possible. But if the psychic being is very conscious, sufficiently conscious, it will seek the light of aspiration in a precise place, because of the culture, the education it will find there. This happens much more frequently than one believes, especially in somewhat educated circles. An intelligent woman with some artistic or philosophical culture, a beginning of conscious individuality, may aspire that the child she is going to have may be the best possible according to her idea or according to what she has read.

1 March 1951

Incarnation in a Particular Body

Mother, when a body is formed, is the soul which incarnates in it compelled to incarnate in that body?

I don't understand your question very well.

The formation of the body depends entirely on a man and a woman, but is the soul which manifests in the child, in the body which is being formed, compelled to manifest in this body?

You mean whether it can choose between different bodies?

Yes.

Well, it is very exceptional, after all, in the great mass of humanity, that a conscious soul incarnates voluntarily. It is something very unusual. I have already told you that when a soul is conscious, fully formed, and wants to incarnate, usually from its psychic plane it looks for a corresponding psychic light at a certain place upon earth. Besides, during its previous incarnation, before going away, before leaving the earth-atmosphere, usually as a result of the experience it had in the life that is coming to an end, the soul chooses more or less — not in all details but broadly — the conditions of its future life. But these are exceptional cases. Possibly we could speak of it for ourselves here, but for the majority, the vast majority of men, even those who are educated, it is out of the question. And what comes then is a psychic being in formation, more or less formed, and there are all the stages of formation from the spark which becomes a little light to the fully formed being, and this extends over thousands of years. This ascent of the soul to become a conscious being having its own will, capable of determining the choice of its own life, takes thousands of years.

So, you are thinking of a soul which would say, "No, I refuse this body, I am going to look for another"?... I don't say it is impossible — everything is possible. It does happen, in fact, that children are still-born, which means that there was no soul to incarnate in them. But it may be for other reasons also; it may be for reasons of malformation only; one can't say. I don't say it is impossible, but generally, when a conscious and free soul chooses to take a body on earth again, even before its birth it works on this body. So it has no reason not to accept even the inconveniences which may result from the ignorance of the parents; for it has chosen the place for a reason which was not one of ignorance: it saw a light there — it might have been simply the light of a possibility, but there was a light and *that* is *why* it has come there. So, it is all very well to say, "Ah! no, I don't like it", but where would it go to choose another it likes?... That may happen, I don't say it is impossible, but it cannot happen very often. For, when from the psychic plane the soul looks at the earth and chooses the place for its next birth, it chooses it with sufficient discernment not to be alto-gether grossly mistaken.

It has also happened that souls have incarnated and then left. There are many reasons why they go away. Children who die very young, after a few days or a few weeks — this may be for a similar reason. Most often it is said that the soul needed just a little experience to complete its formation, that it had it during these few weeks and then left. Everything is possible. And as many stories would be needed to tell the story of souls as are needed to tell the story of men. That is to say, they are innumerable and the instances are as different as possible from one another.

27 June 1956

The Physical Body Is Formed by the Parents

I spoke to you about birth: how souls enter a body; and I told you that the body is formed in a very unsatisfactory way for almost everyone — exceptions are so rare that one can hardly speak of them.

I told you that due to this obscure birth one arrives with a whole physical baggage of things which generally have to be got rid of, if one truly wants to progress, and someone has quoted my own sentence which runs like this:

"You are brought here by force, the environment is imposed on you by force, the laws of atavism of the milieu by force..."

And now the person who wrote to me has asked me who does all that.

Of course I could have been more explicit, but I thought I had been clear enough.

The body is formed by a man and a woman who become the father and mother, and it is they who don't even have the *means* of asking the being they are going to bring into the world whether it would like to come or whether this is in accordance with its destiny. And it is on this body they have formed that they impose by force, by force of necessity, an atavism, an environment, later an education, which will almost always be obstacles to its future growth.

Therefore, I said here and I am repeating it — I thought I had been clear enough — that it was about the physical parents and the physical body I was speaking, nothing else. And that the soul which incarnates, whether it be in course of development or fully developed, has to struggle against the circumstances imposed on it by this animal birth, struggle in order to find its true path and again discover its own self fully. That's all.

27 June 1956

The Soul Will Have to Struggle

Even in the best cases, even when the soul has come consciously, even when it has consciously participated in the formation of the physical body, still so long as the body is formed in the usual animal way, it will have to struggle and correct all those things which come from this human animality.

Inevitably, parents have a particular formation, they are particularly healthy or unhealthy; even taking things at their best, they have a heap of atavisms, habits, formations in the subconscious and even in the unconscious, which come from their own birth, the environment they have lived in, their own life; and even if they are remarkable people, they have a large number of things which are quite opposed to the true psychic life — even the best of them, even the most conscious. And besides, there is all that is going to happen. Even if one takes a great deal of trouble over the education of one's children, they will come in contact with all sorts of people who will have an influence over them, especially when they are very young, and these influences enter the subconscious, one has to struggle against them later on. I say: even in the best cases, because of the way in which the body is formed at present, you have to face innumerable difficulties which come more or less from the subconscious, but rise to the surface and against which you have to struggle before you can become completely free and develop normally.

27 June 1956

The Parents' State of Consciousness

Some children are wicked. Is it because their parents did not aspire for them?

It is perhaps a subconscious wickedness in the parents. It is said that people throw out their wickedness from themselves by giving it birth in their children. One has always a shadow in oneself. There are people who project this outside — that does not always free them from it, but still perhaps it comforts them! But it is the child who "profits" by it, don't you see? It is quite evident that the state of consciousness in which the parents are at that moment is of capital importance. If they have very low and vulgar ideas, the children will reflect them quite certainly. And all these children who are ill-formed, ill-bred, incomplete (specially from the point of view of intelligence: with holes, things missing), children who are only half-conscious and half-formed — this is always due to the fault of the state of consciousness in which the parents were when they conceived the child. Even as the state of consciousness of the last moments of life is of capital importance for the future of the one who is departing, so too the state of consciousness in which the parents are at the moment of conception gives a sort of stamp to the child, which it will reflect throughout its life. So, these are apparently such little things — the mood of the moment, the moment's aspiration or degradation, anything whatsoever, everything that takes place at a particular moment — it seems to be so small a thing, and it has so great a consequence: it brings into the world a child who is incomplete or wicked or finally a failure. And people are not aware of that.

Later, when the child behaves nastily, they scold it. But they should begin by scolding themselves, telling themselves: "In what a horrible state of consciousness must I have been when I brought that child into the world." For it is truly that.

30 December 1953

2

YOUTH, OLD AGE AND DEATH

Youth: The Faculty to Progress

I salute you, my brave little soldiers, I give you my call to the rendez-vous with Victory.

*

My little ones, you are the hope, you are the future. Keep always this youth which is the faculty to progress; for you the phrase "it is impossible" will have no meaning.

*

Remain young, never stop striving towards perfection.

*

For a happy and effective life, the essentials are sincerity, humility, perseverance and an insatiable thirst for progress. Above all one must be convinced of a limitless possibility of progress. Progress is youth; at a hundred years of age one can be young.

*

If the growth of consciousness were considered as the principal goal of life, many difficulties would find their solution. The best way of not becoming old is to make progress the goal of our life.

*

From the moment you are satisfied and aspire no longer, you begin to die. Life is movement, life is effort; it is marching forward, climbing towards future revelations and realisations. Nothing is more dangerous than wanting to rest.

*

Only those years that are passed uselessly make you grow old.

A year spent uselessly is a year during which no progress has been accomplished, no growth in consciousness has been achieved, no further step has been taken towards perfection.

Consecrate your life to the realisation of something higher and broader than yourself and you will never feel the weight of the passing years.

*

Why are men obliged to leave the body?

Because they do not know how to keep up with Nature in her progress towards the Divine.

*

From the viewpoint of the spiritual knowledge decay and dissolution, disintegration are simply, undoubtedly, the result of a wrong attitude.

*

When the body will have learnt the art of ever progressing towards a growing perfection, one will have gone a long way towards conquering the fatality of death.

*

To know how to be reborn into a new life at every moment is the secret of eternal youth.

Youth

Youth does not depend on the small number of years one has lived, but on the capacity to grow and progress. To grow is to increase one's potentialities, one's capacities; to progress is to make constantly more perfect the capacities that one already possesses. Old age does not come from a great number of years but from the incapacity or the refusal to continue to grow and progress. I have known old people of twenty and young people of seventy. As soon as one wants to settle down in life and reap the benefits of one's past efforts, as soon as one thinks that one has done what one had to do and accomplished what one had to accomplish, in short, as soon as one ceases to progress, to advance along the road of perfection, one is sure to fall back and become old.

One can also teach the body that there is almost no limit to its growth in capacities or its progress, provided that one discovers the true method and the right conditioning. This is one of the many experiments which we want to attempt in order to break these collective suggestions and show the world that human potentialities exceed all imagination.

2 February 1949

Old People Who Are Young

There is an old age much more dangerous and much more real than the amassing of years: the incapacity to grow and progress. . . .

As soon as you stop advancing, as soon as you stop progressing, as soon as you cease to better yourself, cease to gain and grow, cease to transform yourself, you truly become old, that is to say, you go downhill towards disintegration.

There are young people who are old and there are old people who are young. If you carry in you this flame for progress and transformation, if you are ready to leave everything behind so that you may advance with an alert step, if you are always open to a new progress, a new improvement, a new transformation, then you are eternally young. But if you sit back satisfied with what has been accomplished, if you have the feeling that you have reached your goal and you have nothing left to do but enjoy the fruit of your efforts, then already more than half your body is in the tomb: it is decrepitude and the true death.

Everything that has been done is always nothing compared with what remains to be done.

Do not look behind. Look ahead, always ahead and go forward always.

25 April 1958

What Makes You Grow Old?

It is not the number of years you have lived that makes you old. You become old when you stop progressing.

As soon as you feel you have done what you had to do, as soon as you think you know what you ought to know, as soon as you want to sit and enjoy the results of your effort, with the feeling you have worked enough in life, then at once you become old and begin to decline.

When, on the contrary, you are convinced that what you know is nothing compared to all that remains to be known, when you feel that what you have done is just the starting-point of what remains to be done, when you see the future like an attractive sun shining with the innumerable possibilities yet to be achieved, then you are young, howsoever many are the years you have passed upon earth, young and rich with all the realisations of tomorrow.

And if you do not want your body to fail you, avoid wasting your energies in useless agitation. Whatever you do, do it in a quiet and composed poise. In peace and silence is the greatest strength.

21 February 1968

Why Physical Progress Stops

All the while you externalise yourself and all the while you bring back something from this externalisation; it is like something porous: a force goes out and then a force comes in. There are pulsations like that. And this is why it is so important to choose the environment in which one lives, because there is constantly a kind of interchange between what you give and what you receive. People who throw themselves out a great deal in activity, receive more. But they receive on the same level, the level of their activity. Children, for example, who are younger, who always move about, always shout and romp and jump (very rarely do they keep quiet, except while asleep, and perhaps not even so), well, they spend much and and they receive much, and generally it is the physical and vital energy that is spent and it is physical and vital energies that are received. They recuperate a good part of what they spend. So there, it is very important for them to be in surroundings where they can, after they have spent or while they are spending, recover something that is at least equal in quality to theirs, that is not of an inferior quality.

When you no longer have this generosity in your movements, you receive much less and this is one of the reasons — one of the chief reasons — why physical progress stops. It is because you become thrifty, you try not to waste; the mind intervenes: "Take care, don't tire yourself, don't do too much, etc." The mind intervenes and physical receptivity diminishes a great deal. Finally, you do not grow any more — by growing reasonable, you stop growing altogether!

5 August 1953

Mental Activity Tends to Paralyse

How is it that as mental activities increase, the capacity to renew one's energies diminishes?

In adults mental activity tends to paralyse the spontaneous movement of exchange of energies. Till he is fourteen, every child, apart from a few rare exceptions, is a little animal; he renews his energies spontaneously like an animal by means of the same activities and exchanges. But the mind introduces a disequilibrium in the being; spontaneous action is replaced by something that wants to know, to regulate, to decide, etc., and to get back this capacity to renew spontaneously one's energies, one must rise to a higher rung above the instincts, that is, from ordinary mental activity one must pass direct into intuition.

25 December 1950

The Receptivity of the Body Is Limited

"In the body the transforming power of Yoga is operative only to a certain degree; for the receptivity of the body is limited. The most material plane of the universe is still in a condition in which receptivity is mixed with a large

amount of resistance. But rapid progress in one part of the being which is not followed by an equivalent progress in other parts produces a disharmony in the nature, a dislocation somewhere; and wherever or whenever this dislocation occurs, it can translate itself into an illness. The nature of the illness depends upon the nature of the dislocation."

The Mother, Questions and Answers 1929

Why is the receptivity of the body limited?

Because in the physical world, in order that things do not get mixed up, it was necessary that it should be somewhat fixed. If, for example, your body were so subtle and plastic that suddenly it began to melt just like that, in the presence of another person, it would be quite annoying! Or when you come nearer, if both were to get mixed up, it would be rather unpleasant! So, because of this, there was a greater concentration, a kind of fixity in the force to separate (it is indeed for the sake of separating) one individuality from another. And this fixity is just what prevents the body from progressing as rapidly as it could and should. And as one grows up and reaches one's normal height and constitution, one becomes still more rigid. For children have this plasticity of growth, they are changing all the time, they are visibly changing. Therefore so long as they are young and are growing and developing, they have a certain plasticity in them, but when you are over forty and as generally in life you then sit down and think that you have reached your goal and are about to gather the fruit of your labour, you become dry and hard like wood and even like stone in the end. And as the body is no longer able to adapt itself to the movement of inner transformation, it drags, it ages and cannot keep pace any more, it dries up. . . .

Is it not possible, by yogic force, to prevent the body from being rigid?

It is possible. When you do gymnastics, is it not to make your body less rigid? And you go on progressing: what you cannot do the first year, you are able to do after a few years. There are people who obtain an almost total suppleness, those, for example, who do Asanas. Yes, one can obtain almost complete suppleness. But an ordinary man, if he tried to do these exercises, would break something in him. Well, it happens like that. With the mind, it is the same thing. It is through gymnastic exercises that you make yourself supple. It is a question of discipline, of development. . . .

You have said that on the material plane "receptivity is mixed with a large amount of resistance." What is this resistance?

Don't you have resistances in your body, don't you? When you want to do an exercise, can you do with your body whatever you want? And when you try to be in good health, does your body always obey? And when you want to learn your lesson, does your brain follow it without difficulty?... That is the resistance, it is all that refuses to progress. And I believe that unfortunately the amount of resistance is much greater than the amount of receptivity. One must work very hard to become receptive.

16 September 1953

The Incapacity of the Body

It is just because progress is not constant and perpetual in the physical world that there is a growth, an apogee, a decline and a decomposition. For anything that does not advance, falls back; all that does not progress, regresses.

So this is just what happens physically. The physical world has not learnt how to progress indefinitely; it arrives at a certain point, then it is either tired of progressing or is not capable of progressing in the present constitution, but in any case it stops progressing and after a time decomposes. . . .

It is the incapacity of the body to transform itself, to continue progressing that causes it to regress and in the end become more and more open to the inner disequilibrium until one day that becomes strong enough to bring about a total imbalance and it can no longer regain its balance and health.

5 August 1953

The Body Decays, Declines

*If men did not die, with age their body would be-
come useless?*

Ah! No. You are looking from the wrong side. They could escape dying only if their body did not decay. It is just because their body decays that they die. It is because their body becomes useless that they die. If they are not to die, their body should not become useless. This is just the contrary. It is precisely because the body decays, declines and ends in a complete degradation that death becomes necessary. But if the body followed the progressive movement of the inner being, if it had the same sense of progress and perfection as the psychic being, there would be no necessity for it to die. One year added to another need not bring a deterioration. It is only a habit of Nature. It is only a habit of what is happening at *this* moment. And that is exactly the cause of death. One can foresee quite well, on the contrary, that the movement for perfection which is at the beginning of life might continue under another form. I have already told you that one does not foresee an uninterrupted growth, for that would need changing the height of the houses after some time! But this growth in height may be changed into a growth in perfection: the perfection of the form. All the imperfections of the form may be gradually corrected, all the weaknesses replaced by strength, all the incapacities by skill. Why should it not be like this? You do not think in that way because you have the habit of seeing things otherwise. But there is no reason why this should not happen. . . .

One sheds off something, but it's in order to grow again and have something more. One must be able to keep the harmony and the beauty till the end. There is no reason why one should have a body which has no longer any purpose in being, in existing; because it would no longer be good for anything. To be no longer good for anything, that is exactly what makes it disappear. One could have a body that grows from perfection to perfection. There are many things in the body that make you say: "Ah, if it were like that! Ah, I would like it to be thus!" (I am not speaking of your character, for there are so many things that need changing; I am speaking only of your physical appearance). You see some disharmony somewhere and you say: "If this disharmony disappeared, how much better would it be!"... But why don't you think that it could be done? If you look at yourself in quite an objective way — not with that sort of attachment one has for one's little person, but quite objectively, you look at yourself as you would look at another person and tell yourself: "But this thing is not altogether in harmony with that", and if you look yet more closely, it becomes very interesting: you discover that this disharmony is the expression of a defect in your character. It is because in your character there is something a bit twisted, not quite harmonious, and in your body this is reproduced somewhere. You try to arrange it in your body and you find out that to get back to the source of this physical disharmony, you have to find out the defect in your inner being. And then you begin to work and the result is obtained.

You don't know to what an extent the body is plastic! From another standpoint, I would say it is terribly rigid and that is why the body deteriorates. But that is because we do not know how to make use of it. We do not know, when we are still fresh like little leaves, how to will for a luxuriant, magnificent, faultless flowering. And instead of telling oneself with a somewhat miserable look: "It is a pity my arms are too thin or my legs are too long or my back is not straight or my head is not quite harmonious", if one said: "It must be otherwise, my arms must be proportionate, my body harmonious, every form in me must express a higher beauty", then one will succeed. And you will succeed if you know how to do it with the true will that is persistent, tranquil, that is not impatient, does not care for appearances of defeat, continues its work quietly, very quietly, continues to will that it be so, to look for the inner reason, to discover it, to work with energy. Immediately, as soon as you see a little black worm somewhere, which does not look pretty and makes a small rather unpleasant, disgusting stain, you pick it up, pull it out and throw it away and put a lovely light in its place. And after a time you discover: "Why! that disharmony I had in my face is disappearing; that sign of brutality, unconsciousness which was in my expression, it is going away." And then ten years later you don't recognise yourself any longer.

You are all, here, youthful matter; you must know how to profit by it — and not for petty, selfish and stupid reasons but for the love of beauty, for the need of harmony.

If the body is to last, it must not deteriorate. There must not be any decay. It must win on one side: it must be a transformation, it must not be a decay. With decay there is no possibility of immortality.

17 June 1953

"No, I Will Not Die"

Sometimes when people are dying, they know that they are about to die. Why don't they tell the spirit [of death] to go away?

Ah! well, it depends upon the people. Two things are necessary. First of all, nothing in your being, no part of your being should want to die. That does not happen often. You have always a defeatist in you somewhere: something that is tired, something that is disgusted, something that has had enough of it, something that is lazy, something that does not want to struggle and says: "Well! Ah! Let it be finished, so much the better." That is sufficient, you are dead.

But it is a fact: if nothing, absolutely nothing in you consents to die, you will not die. For someone to die, there is always a second, perhaps the hundredth part of a second when he gives his consent. If there is not this second of consent, he does not die.

I knew people who should have really died according to all physical and vital laws; and they refused. They said: "No,

I will not die", and they lived. There are others who do not need at all to die, but they are of that kind and say: "Ah! Well! Yes, so much the better, it will be finished", and it is finished. Even that much, even nothing more than that: you need not have a persistent wish, you have only to say: "Well, yes, I have had enough!" and it is finished. So it is truly like that. As you say, you may have death standing by your bedside and tell him: "I do not want you, go away", and it will be obliged to go away. But usually one gives way, for one must struggle, one must be strong, one must be very courageous and enduring, must have a great faith in the necessity of life; like someone, for example, who feels very strongly that he has still something to do and he must absolutely do it. But who is sure he has not within him the least bit of a defeatist, somewhere, who just yields and says: "It is all right"?... It is here, the necessity of unifying oneself.

1 July 1953

Make Death Magnificent

If one must for some reason or other leave one's body and take a new one, is it not better to make of one's death something magnificent, joyful, enthusiastic, than to make it a disgusting defeat? Those who cling on, who try by every possible means to delay the end even by a minute or two, who give you an example of frightful anguish, show that they are not conscious of their soul.... After all, it is perhaps a means, isn't it? One can change this accident into a means; if one is conscious one can make a beautiful thing of it, a very beautiful thing, as of everything. And note, those who do not fear it, who are not anxious, who can die without any sordidness are those who never think about it, who are not haunted all the time by this "horror" facing them which they must escape and which they try to push as far away from them as they can. These, when the occasion comes, can lift their head, smile and say, "Here I am."

It is they who have the will to make the best possible use of their life, it is they who say, "I shall remain here as long as it is necessary, to the last second, and I shall not lose one moment to realise my goal"; these, when the necessity comes, put up the best show. Why? — It is very simple, because they live in their ideal, the truth of their ideal; because that is the real thing for them, the very reason of their being, and in all things they can see this ideal, this reason of existence, and never do they come down into the sordidness of material life.

So, the conclusion:

One must never wish for death.

One must never will to die.

One must never be afraid to die.

And in all circumstances one must will to exceed oneself.

23 April 1951

3

TRANSFORMATION

The Work of Transformation

Of all things the most difficult is to bring down the Divine Consciousness into the material world; must the endeavour be abandoned on that account! Surely not.

*

There is a Supreme Divine Consciousness. We want to manifest this Divine Consciousness in the physical life.

*

The goal is not to lose oneself in the Divine Consciousness. The goal is to let the Divine Consciousness penetrate into Matter and transform it.

*

The spirituality of tomorrow will take up matter and transform it.

*

Immortality is not a goal, it is not even a means. It will proceed naturally from the fact of living the Truth.

*

The target at which we are aiming is immortality. And of all habits, death is surely the most obstinate.

*

Unless one has an endless patience and an unshakable perseverance, it is better not to start on the way of transformation.

*

Somebody asked me, —

"In the work of Transformation, who is the slowest to do his part, man or God?"

I replied, —

Man finds that God is too slow to answer his prayers.

God finds that man is too slow to receive His influence.

But for the Truth-Consciousness all is going on as it ought to go.

An Integral Transformation

We want an integral transformation, the transformation of the body and all its activities.

Formerly, when one spoke of transformation one meant solely the transformation of the inner consciousness. One tried to discover in oneself this deep consciousness and rejected the body and its activities like an encumbrance and a useless thing, in order to attend only to the inner movement. Sri Aurobindo declared that this was not enough; the Truth demanded that the material world should also participate in the transformation and become an expression of the deeper Truth. But when people heard this, many thought that it was possible to transform the body and its activities without bothering in the least about what was happening within — naturally this is not quite true. Before you can undertake this work of physical transformation, which of all things is the most difficult, your inner consciousness must be firmly established, solidly established in the Truth, so that this transformation may be the final expression of the Truth — "final" for the moment at least.

The starting-point of this transformation is receptivity, we have already spoken about it. That is the indispensable condition for obtaining the transformation. Then comes the change of consciousness. This change of consciousness and its preparation have often been compared with the formation of the chicken in the egg: till the very last second the egg remains the same, there is no change, and it is only when the chicken is completely formed, absolutely alive, that it itself makes with its little beak a hole in the shell and comes out. Something similar takes place at the moment of the change of consciousness. For a long time you have the impression that nothing is happening, that your consciousness is the same as usual, and, if you have an intense aspiration, you even feel a resistance, as though you were knocking against a wall which does not yield. But when you are ready within, a last effort — the pecking in the shell of the being — and everything opens and you are projected into another consciousness.

I said that it was a revolution of the basic equilibrium, that is, a total reversal of consciousness comparable with what happens to light when it passes through a prism. Or it is as though you were turning a ball inside out, which cannot be done except in the fourth dimension. One comes out of the ordinary three-dimensional consciousness to enter the higher four-dimensional consciousness, and into an infinite number of dimensions. This is the indispensable starting-point. Unless your consciousness changes its dimension, it will remain just what it is with the superficial vision of things, and all the profundities will escape you.

4 January 1951

The Physical Battle

We come now to the most terrible battle of all, the physical battle which is fought in the body; for it goes on without respite or truce. It begins at birth and can end only with the defeat of one of the two combatants: the force of transformation and the force of disintegration. I say at birth, for in fact the two movements are in conflict from the very moment one comes into the world, although the conflict becomes conscious and deliberate only much later. For every indisposition, every illness, every malformation, even accidents, are the result of the action of the force of disintegration, just as growth, harmonious development, resistance to attack, recovery from illness, every return to the normal functioning, every progressive improvement, are due to the action of the force of transformation. Later on, with the development of the consciousness, when the fight becomes deliberate, it changes into a frantic race between the two opposite and rival movements, a race to see which one will reach its goal first, transformation or death. This means a ceaseless effort, a constant concentration to call down the regenerating force and to increase the receptivity of the cells to this force, to fight step by step, from point to point against the devastating action of the forces of destruction and decline, to tear out of its grasp everything that is capable of responding to the ascending urge, to enlighten, purify and stabilise. It is an obscure and obstinate struggle, most often without any apparent result or any external sign of the partial victories that have been won and are ever uncertain — for the work that has been done always seems to need to be redone; each step forward is most often made at the cost of a setback elsewhere and what has been done one day can be undone the next. Indeed, the victory can be sure and lasting only when it is total. And all that takes time, much time, and the years pass by inexorably, increasing the strength of the adverse forces.

All this time the consciousness stands like a sentinel in a trench: you must hold on, hold on at all costs, without a quiver of fear or a slackening of vigilance, keeping an unshakable faith in the mission to be accomplished and in the help from above which inspires and sustains you. For the victory will go to the most enduring.

Bulletin, *February 1954*

This Movement of Progressive Harmony

By means of a rational and discerning physical education, we must make our body strong and supple enough to become a fit instrument in the material world for the truth-force which wants to manifest through us.

In fact, the body must not rule, it must obey. By its very nature it is a docile and faithful servant. Unfortunately, it rarely has the capacity of discernment it ought to have with regard to its masters, the mind and the vital. It obeys them blindly, at the cost of its own well-being. The mind with its dogmas, its rigid and arbitrary principles, the vital with its passions, its excesses and dissipations soon destroy the natural balance of the body and create in it fatigue, exhaustion and disease. It must be freed from this tyranny and this can be done only through a constant union with the psychic centre of the being. The body has a wonderful capacity of adaptation and endurance. It is able to do many more things than one usually imagines. If, instead of the ignorant and despotic masters that now govern it, it is ruled by the central truth of the being, you will be amazed at what it is capable of doing. Calm and quiet, strong and poised, at every minute it will be able to put forth the effort that is demanded of it, for it will have learnt to find rest in action and to recuperate, through contact with the universal forces, the energies it expends consciously and usefully. In this sound and balanced life a new harmony will manifest in the body, reflecting the harmony of the higher regions, which will give it perfect proportions and ideal beauty of form. And this harmony will be progressive, for the truth of the being is never static; it is a perpetual unfolding of a growing perfection that is more and more total and comprehensive. As soon as the body has learnt to follow this movement of progressive harmony, it will be possible for it to escape, through a continuous process of transformation, from the necessity of disintegration and destruction. Thus the irrevocable law of death will no longer have any reason to exist.

Bulletin, *November 1950*

The ABC of the Transformation of the Body

Now, as you know, from the physical point of view human beings live in frightful ignorance. They cannot even say exactly... For instance, would you be able to tell exactly, at every meal, the amount of food and the kind of food your body needs? — simply that, nothing more than that: how much should be taken and when it should be taken. . . . You know nothing about it, there's just a vague idea of it, a sort of imagination or guesswork or deduction or... all sorts of things which have nothing to do with knowledge. But that exact knowledge: "This is what I must eat, I must eat this much" — and then it is finished. "This my body needs." Well, that can be done. There's a time when one knows it very well. But it asks for years of labour, and above all years of work almost without any mental control, just with a consciousness that's subtle enough to establish a connection with the elements of transformation and progress. And to know also how to determine for one's body, exactly, the amount of physical effort, of material activity, of expenditure and recuperation of energy, the proportion between what is received and what is given, the utilisation of energies to re-establish a state of equilibrium, which has been broken, to make the cells which are lagging behind progress, to build conditions for the possibility of higher progress, etc... it is a formidable task. And yet, it is that which must be done if one hopes to transform one's body. First it must be put completely in harmony with the inner consciousness. And to do that, it is a work in each cell, so to say, in each little activity, in every movement of the organs. With this alone one could be busy day and night without having to do anything else. . . . One does not keep up the effort and, above all, the concentration, nor the inner vision.

I have put to you quite a superficial question: it seems astonishing to you that one can know the exact amount of what one should eat, and what should be eaten at a certain time, and at what time one should take one's meal, and when one is ready for another! Well, that is an altogether superficial part of the problem, yet if you enter into the combination of the cells and the inner organisation in order that all this may be ready to respond to the descending Force. . . First, are you conscious of your physical cells and their different characteristics, their activity, the degree of their receptivity, of what is in a healthy condition and what is not? Can you say with certainty when you are tired, why you are tired? When there's something wrong somewhere, can you say, "It is because of this that I am suffering"?... Why do people rush to the doctor? Because they are under the illusion that the doctor knows better than they how to look inside their body and find out what's going on there — which is not very reasonable, but still that's the habit!

But for oneself, who can look inside himself quite positively and precisely and know exactly what is out of order, why it is disturbed, how it has been disturbed? And all this is simply a work of observation; afterwards one must do what is necessary to put it back into order again, and that is still more difficult.

Well, this is the ABC of the transformation of the body. *Voilà*.

24 February 1954

Endless Patience and Endurance

One must be careful, . . . one must not say, "Here we are, it's no use, I shall never achieve anything, all my efforts are futile; all this is an illusion, it is impossible." On the contrary, one must say, "I wasn't vigilant enough." One must wait long, very long, before one can say, "Ah! it is done and finished." Sometimes one must wait for years, many years....

I am not saying this to discourage you, but to give you patience and perseverance — for there is a moment when you do arrive. And note that the vital is a small part of your being — a very important part, we have said that it is the dynamism, the realising energy, it is very important; but it is only a small part. And the mind!... which goes wandering, which must be pulled back by all the strings to be kept quiet! You think this can be done overnight? And your body?... You have a weakness, a difficulty, sometimes a small chronic illness, nothing much, but still it is a nuisance, isn't it? You want to get rid of it. You make efforts, you concentrate; you work upon it, establish harmony, and you think it is finished, and then... Take, for instance, people who have the habit of coughing; they can't control themselves or almost can't. It is not serious but it is bothersome, and there seems to be no reason why it should ever stop. Well, one tells oneself, "I am going to control this." One makes an effort — a yogic effort, not a material one — one brings down consciousness, force, and stops the cough. And one thinks, "The body has forgotten how to cough." And it is a great thing when the body has forgotten; truly one can say, "I am cured." But unfortunately it is not always true, for this goes down into the subconscient and, one day, when the balance of forces is not so well established, when the strength is not the same, it begins again. And one laments, "I believed that it was over! I had succeeded and told myself, 'It is true that spiritual power has an action upon the body, it is true that something can be done', and there! It is not true. And yet it was a small thing, and I who want to conquer immortality! How will I succeed?... For years I have been free from this small thing and here it is beginning anew!" It is then that you must be careful.

You must arm yourself with an endless patience and endurance. You do a thing once, ten times, a hundred times, a thousand times if necessary, but you do it till it gets done. And not done only here and there, but everywhere and everywhere at the same time.

26 March 1951

A Total Conversion Is Necessary

Until now all the victories which have been won have reactions that are finally defeats. There is never anything definitive and complete. Every time one has the feeling of having gained a victory, one finds out that this victory was incomplete, partial, fugitive. This is a fact one can always observe if one looks carefully at oneself. Not that things are necessarily what they were before, no, something has changed, but everything has not changed and not changed completely.

This is very apparent, very noticeable in physical conquests over the body. Through a very assiduous labour one succeeds in overcoming a weakness, a limitation, a bad habit, and one believes this is a definitive victory; but after some time or at times immediately, one realises that nothing is completely done, nothing is definitive, that what one thought to be accomplished has to be done again. For only a total change of consciousness and the intervention of a new force, a reversal of consciousness can make the victory complete.

In the old Chaldean tradition, very often the young novices were given an image when they were invested with the white robe; they were told: "Do not try to remove the stains one by one, the whole robe must be purified." Do not try to correct your faults one by one, to overcome your weaknesses one by one, it does not take you very far. The entire consciousness must be changed, a reversal of consciousness must be achieved, a springing up out of the state in which one is towards a higher state from which one dominates all the weaknesses one wants to heal, and from which one has a full vision of the work to be accomplished.

I believe Sri Aurobindo has said this: things are such that it may be said that nothing is done until everything is done. One step ahead is not enough, a total conversion is necessary.

How many times have I heard people who were making an effort say, "I try, but what's the use of my trying? Every time I think I have gained something, I find that I must begin all over again." This happens because they are trying to go forward while standing still, they are trying to progress without changing their consciousness. It is the entire point of view which must be shifted, the whole consciousness must get out of the rut in which it lies so as to rise up and see things from above. It is only thus that victories will not be changed into defeats.

26 December 1956

A SKETCH OF THE MOTHER'S LIFE

Originally named Mirra Alfassa, the Mother was born in Paris on 21 February 1878. She was the daughter of Maurice Alfassa, a banker (born in Adrianople, Turkey in 1843) and Mathilde Ismaloun (born in Alexandria, Egypt in 1857). Maurice, his wife and his son, Mattéo (born in Alexandria in 1876), emigrated from Egypt to France in 1877, one year before Mirra's birth. Her early education was given at home. Around 1892 she attended a studio to learn drawing and painting, and later studied at the École de Beaux Arts. Her paintings were exhibited at the Paris Salon.

Concerning her early spiritual life, the Mother has written: "Between 11 and 13 a series of psychic and spiritual experiences revealed to me not only the existence of God but man's possibility of uniting with Him, of realising Him integrally in consciousness and action, of manifesting Him upon earth in a life divine." In her late twenties the Mother voyaged to Tlemcen, Algeria, where she studied occultism for two years with a Polish adept, Max Théon, and his wife. Returning to Paris in 1906, she founded her first group of spiritual seekers. She gave many talks to various groups in Paris between 1911 and 1913.

At the age of thirty-six the Mother journeyed to Pondicherry, India, to meet Sri Aurobindo. She saw him on 29 March 1914 and at once recognised him as the one who for many years had inwardly been guiding her spiritual development. Staying for eleven months, she was obliged to return to France because of the war. She lived in France for about a year and then in Japan for almost four years. On 24 April 1920 she returned to Pondicherry to resume her collaboration with Sri Aurobindo, and remained for the rest of her life.

At that time a small group of disciples had gathered around Sri Aurobindo. The increase of disciples led to the founding of the Sri Aurobindo Ashram on 24 November 1926. From the beginning Sri Aurobindo entrusted the Mother with full material and spiritual charge of the Ashram. Through nearly fifty years of work, she created the community which at present consists of about 2000 persons. This figure includes 530 students who attend the Sri Aurobindo International Centre of Education. This institution, an extension of the Ashram, was inaugurated on 6 January 1952. The first Ashram school opened on 2 December 1943 with only twenty students. Another of the Mother's conceptions was an international township, Auroville, the "City of Dawn", founded on 28 February 1968. About 500 persons from India and other nations now live in Auroville.

The Mother left her body on 17 November 1973, at the age of ninety-five.

GLOSSARY

These definitions are based upon the writings of Sri Aurobindo.

Ananda — bliss, delight, spiritual ecstasy; the essential principle of delight.

Asana — fixed posture; held position of the body.

Force, the — not mental or vital energy but the Divine Force from above; a higher consciousness using its power, a spiritual and supraphysical force acting on the physical world directly.

Inner being — the inner mind, inner vital, inner physical with the psychic behind as the inmost. There are, we might say, two beings in us, one on the surface, our ordinary exterior mind, life, body consciousness, another behind the veil, an inner mind, an inner life, an inner physical consciousness constituting another or inner self.

Mantra — sacred syllable, name or mystic formula; set words or sounds having a spiritual significance and power.

Mind (the mental) — the part of the nature which has to do with cognition and intelligence, with ideas, with mental or thought perceptions, the reactions of thought to things, with the truly mental movements and formations, mental vision and will, etc., that are part of man's intelligence.

Psychic being — the soul of the individual evolving in the manifestation; the soul in the secret heart supporting by its presence the action of the mind, life and body.

Rajas — one of the three qualities or modes of Nature; the mode of passion, action and struggling emotion; the force of kinesis.

Sachchidananda — the trinity of Existence [*sat*], Consciousness [*cit*] and Delight [*ānanda*]; the One with a triple aspect.

Sadhak — one who practises a system of yoga.

Sadhana — method, system, practice of yoga.

Samadhi — trance; yogic trance; ecstatic trance in which the consciousness passes away from outer objects.

Sannyasin — an ascetic; one who has renounced.

Sattwa — one of the three qualities or modes of Nature; the mode of poise, knowledge and satisfaction; the force of equilibrium.

Supramental, the — the Truth-Consciousness, Truth in possession of itself and fulfilling itself by its own power.

Tamas — one of the three qualities or modes of Nature; the mode of ignorance and inertia; the force of inconscience and inertia.

Transformation — means that the higher consciousness or nature is brought down into the mind, vital and body and takes the place of the lower.

Vital, the — the Life-nature made up of desires, sensations, feelings, passions, energies of action, will of desire, reactions of the desire-soul in man and of all that play of possessive and other related instincts, anger, greed, lust, etc., that belong to this field of the nature.

Vital world — a world in which Matter is not supreme, but rather Life-force. Desire and the satisfaction of impulse are the first law of this world of sheer vital existence in which the life-power plays with so much greater a freedom and capacity than in our physical living; it may be called the desire-world, for that is its principal characteristic.

Yoga — joining; union with the Self, the Spirit or the Divine.

REFERENCES

The passages in this book have been selected from the following books and journals published by the Sri Aurobindo Ashram, Pondicherry, India.

COLLECTED WORKS OF THE MOTHER

Vol. 2	Words of Long Ago
Vol. 3	Questions and Answers
Vol. 4	Questions and Answers 1950-51
Vol. 5	Questions and Answers 1953
Vol. 6	Questions and Answers 1954
Vol. 8	Questions and Answers 1956
Vol. 9	Questions and Answers 1957-58
Vol. 10	On Thoughts and Aphorisms
Vol. 12	On Education

BOOKS

Champaklal Speaks, 1975 Edition
Champaklal's Treasures, 1976 Edition
Mantras of the Mother I, 1975 Edition
Words of the Mother I, 1938 Edition
Words of the Mother II, 1949 Edition
Words of the Mother (Enlarged), 1949 Edition

JOURNALS

The Advent
All India Magazine
Bulletin of Sri Aurobindo International Centre of Education
Gazette Aurovilienne
Mother India
Sri Aurobindo Circle